ONE Touch Physiology

For NEET PG/FMGE/INI-CET/Undergraduates

ONE Touch Physiology

For NEET PG/FMGE/INI-CET/Undergraduates

S Krishna Kumar MD

CBSPD
Dedicated to Education

CBS Publishers & Distributors Pvt Ltd

• New Delhi • Bengaluru • Chennai • Kochi • Kolkata • Lucknow • Mumbai
• Hyderabad • Jharkhand • Nagpur • Patna • Pune • Uttarakhand

ONE Touch Physiology

For NEET PG/FMGE/INI-CET/Undergraduates

ISBN: 978-93-94525-60-3

First Edition: 2024

Published by **Satish Kumar Jain** and produced by **Varun Jain** for

CBS Publishers & Distributors Pvt Ltd
4819/XI Prahlad Street, 24 Ansari Road, Daryaganj, New Delhi 110 002, India.
Ph: +91-11-23289259, 23266861, 23266867 Website: www.cbspd.com
Fax: 011-23243014
e-mail: delhi@cbspd.com; cbspubs@airtelmail.in.

Corporate Office: 204 FIE, Industrial Area, Patparganj, Delhi 110 092
Ph: +91-11-4934 4934 Fax: 4934 4935
e-mail: feedback@cbspd.com; bhupesharora@cbspd.com

Branches

- **Bengaluru:** Seema House 2975, 17th Cross, K.R. Road, Banasankari 2nd Stage, Bengaluru-560 070, Karnataka
  Ph: +91-80-26771678/79 Fax: +91-80-26771680 e-mail: bangalore@cbspd.com
- **Chennai:** 7, Subbaraya Street, Shenoy Nagar, Chennai-600 030, Tamil Nadu
  Ph: +91-44-26680620, 26681266 Fax: +91-44-42032115 e-mail: chennai@cbspd.com
- **Kochi:** 68/1534, 35, 36-Power House Road, Opp. KSEB, Cochin-682018, Kochi, Kerala
  Ph: +91-484-4059061-65 Fax: +91-484-4059065 e-mail: kochi@cbspd.com
- **Kolkata:** Hind Ceramics Compound, 1st Floor, 147, Nilganj Road, Belghoria, Kolkata-700056, West Bengal
  Ph: +033-2563-3055/56 e-mail: kolkata@cbspd.com
- **Lucknow:** Basement, Khushnuma Complex, 7-Meerabai Marg (Behind Jawahar Bhawan), Lucknow-226001, Uttar Pradesh
  Ph: +0522-4000032 e-mail: tiwari.lucknow@cbspd.com
- **Mumbai:** PWD Shed, Gala No. 25/26, Ramchandra Bhatt Marg, Next to J.J. Hospital Gate No. 2, Opp. Union Bank of India, Noor Baug, Mumbai-400009, Maharashtra
  Ph: +91-22-66661880/89 Fax: +91-22-24902342 e-mail: mumbai@cbspd.com

Representatives

- **Hyderabad** +91-9885175004
- **Jharkhand** +91-9811541605
- **Nagpur** +91-9421945513
- **Patna** +91-9334159340
- **Pune** +91-9623451994
- **Uttarakhand** +91-9716462459

Printed at : Goyal Offset Works Pvt. Ltd. Haryana

Dedicated to

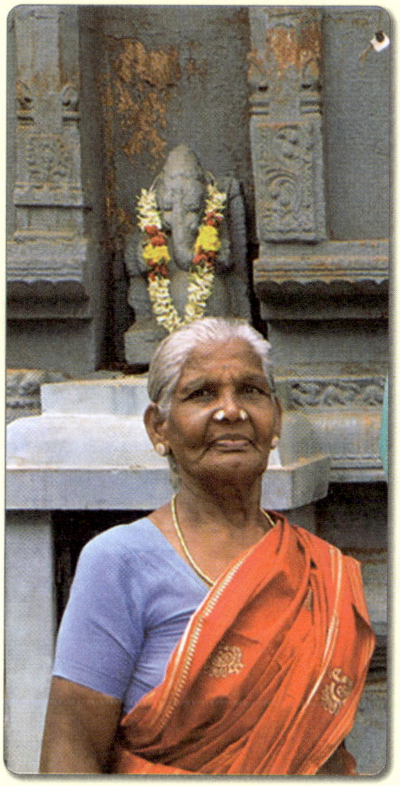

"My Aunt Mrs Subbulakshmi Ammal who took care of me right from my 10 years of age"

Preface

Dear Students,

With immense love and gratitude, I present to you the book "One Touch Physiology". But before you start going through this extremely useful work, it is essential to discuss with you the following specialties of this book:

- **High Yield** is the word. This book is designed in such a way that it helps you to go through all the most important areas you need to remember for your exams.
- **MIMT**: Maximum Information in Minimum Time. This book is loaded with whole lot of important information presented in a concise way so that you can read and revise the entire content in short time.
- **KISS**: Keep It Simple & Significant. The language used while writing this book is simple one so that anybody can easily understand the content. All the complex concepts are simplified.
- **Prime Time Show**: This book is very effective, especially when your exam is round the corner. (Prime time). It will be so handy to you to go through all the important topics just before exams.
- **Revision is the Key**: Perhaps the single most important objective of this book is it helps you to REVISE physiology effectively because important areas are covered concisely in a few pages.
- **See and Learn**: All the important images are given in the book. It helps you to tackle the image-based questions in exams.
- **Tables, Flowcharts & Must Know**: Content is presented in the form of tables and flowcharts for effective reading. Must know areas are highlighted for your convenience.
- **Past Guides Our Future**: All the questions asked in the recent exams are given with answers in this book. Mastering Repeat topics and Repeat questions is an important trait of a successful candidate.

Although I have tried my level best to make this book error free, kindly do let me know in case you come across any errors through my mail ID: tallboykk&gmail.com or through Instagram to my page @ krishnakumar_solaiappan

"All good things will happen at the right time. Have patience. Be well prepared and stay persistent and consistent. Stay hopeful always".

My good luck and best wishes are always there for you!

Yours Lovingly

S Krishna Kumar

Contents

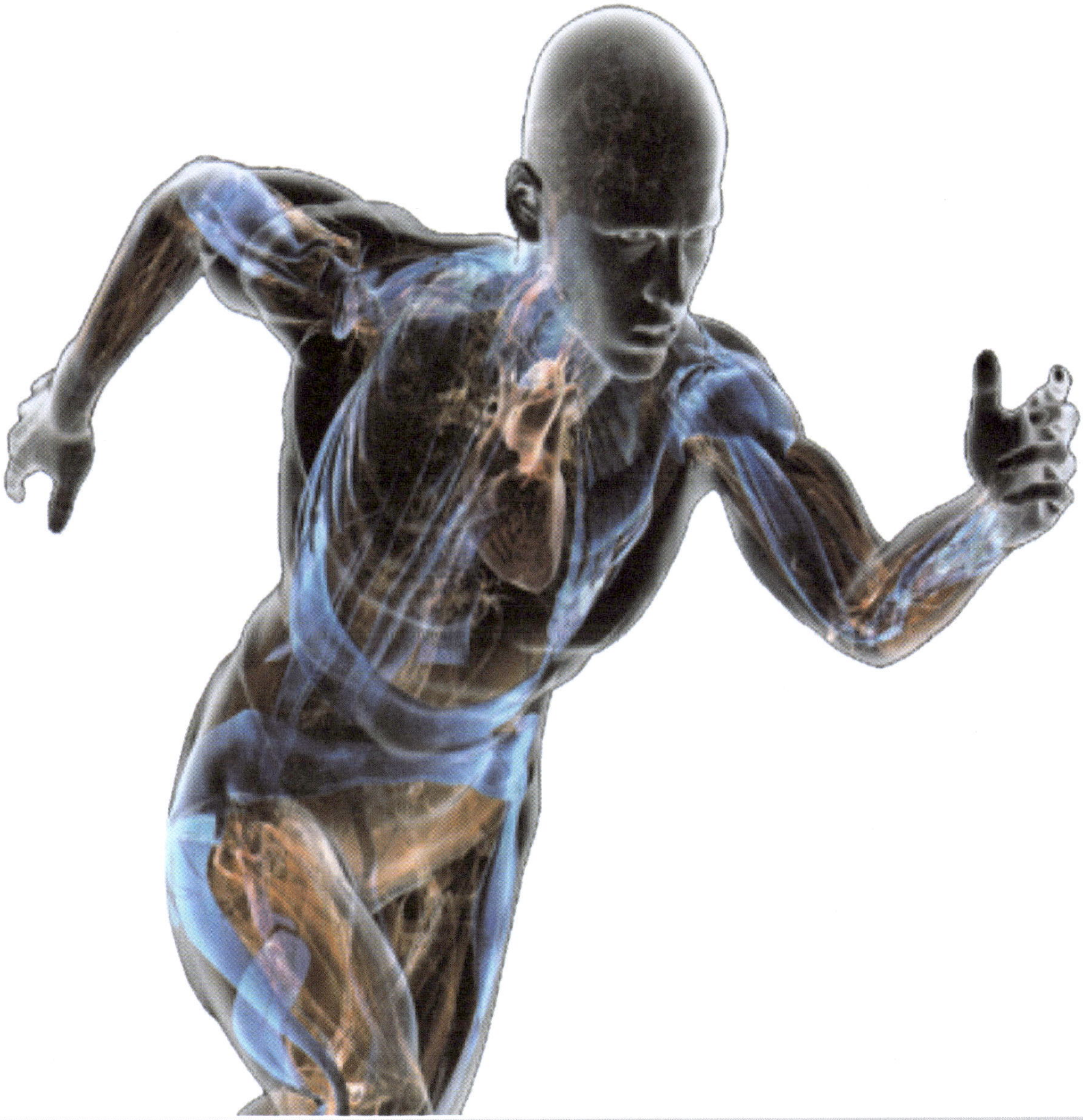

THEORY

1. GENERAL PHYSIOLOGY

HOMEOSTASIS

- All our body parameters must be maintained at **NEAR NORMAL** levels. This concept of **CONSTANCY** is called **HOMEOSTASIS**.
- Dynamic Equilibrium- Constancy of body parameters is maintained under the fluctuating limits (Range). For example, Normal Heart Rate ranges from 60 to 100 beats/min.
- The term Homeostasis was coined by Walter Cannon.
- Body parameters are maintained at constant levels mainly in Extracellular Fluid (ECF).
- This Extracellular Fluid (ECF) is the stable internal environment (milieu interior) for cells.
- Claude Bernard coined the term milieu interior.
- Homeostasis is maintained by **control systems.**
- The control systems are **Negative Feedback, Positive Feedback and Feed Forward Control.**

Control systems

Negative feedback
- Here INCREASED level of that parameter is immediately followed by DECREASE
- Also called **balancing feedback**
- Examples of negative feedback blood pressure regulation by **BAROREFLEX**, Endocrine hormone regulation
- The degree of effectiveness of the negative feedback is determined by GAIN
- The formula for calculating gain is, Gain = Correction/error
- KIDNEY displays **infinite feedback gain** principle in regulation of BP which means it will not leave any error during correction of BP

Positive feedback
- Here INCREASED level of that parameter is immediately followed by further INCREASE
- Positive feedback, once started, it enhances or amplifies the effect on its own. That is why positive feedback is also called VICIOUS CYCLE
- Examples of positive feedback can be easily remembered with this mnemonic CLASP
- Clotting, calcium entry into SR, LH surge, action potential, shock, parturition
- Ferguson reflex—positive feedback reflex is seen during parturition because of oxytocin
- Only time where the endocrine hormone regulation comes under positive feedback is **luteinizing hormone (LH)** surge around ovulation and the hormone responsible is ESTROGEN

Feed forward control
- Here no stimulus is required but still the system ANTICIPATES and makes corrective changes
- Also called **anticipatory or adaptive control**
- Examples of feed forward control are:
  - Temperature control—thermoregulatory responses are initiated by hypothalamus BEFORE the changes in environmental temperature have succeeded in changing the body's core body temperature
  - Cephalic phase of gastric secretion (Just thinking about food increases gastric acid production)
  - Thinking about exercise itself increases heart rate and respiratory rate
  - Role of cerebellum in motor coordination

2. CELLULAR PHYSIOLOGY

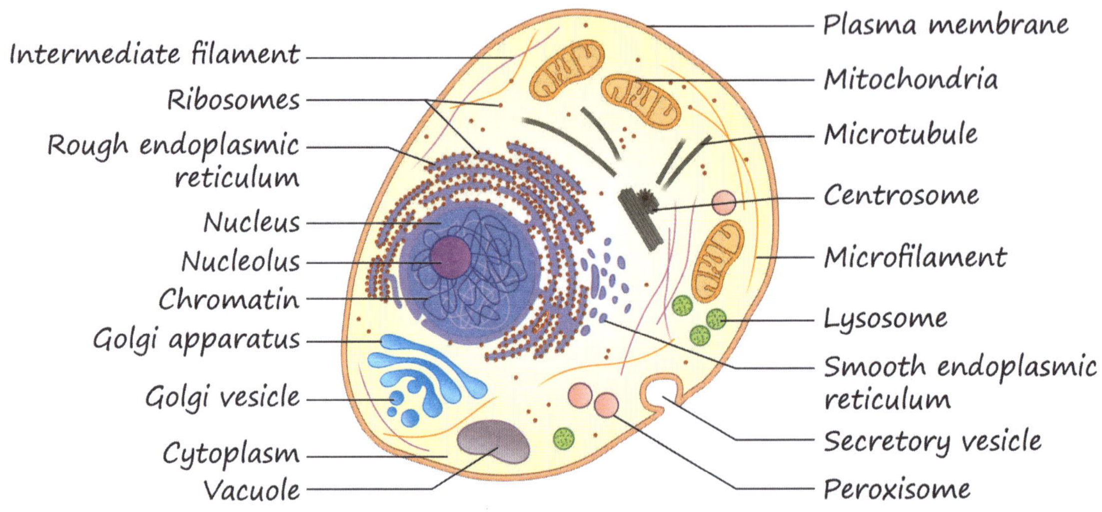

CELL MEMBRANE (PLASMA MEMBRANE)

- It is a selectively permeable barrier.
- Cell membrane contains Lipids (45%), Proteins (55%) and Carbohydrates (5%).
- **Fluid Mosaic Model** proposed by **Singer and Nicholson** explains the components of cell membrane and their functions.
- Proteins are the major constituents of cell membrane.
- Inner mitochondria membrane has maximum protein concentration.
- The only exception where lipids outnumber proteins is myelin sheath of nerve cell membrane.

Membrane Lipids (Fluid Component)

- Three types of lipids are seen in cell membrane—phospholipids, glycolipids and cholesterol.
- Most lipids are distributed unequally (Membrane Asymmetry).

Phospholipids and their characteristics and clinical importance

Phospholipids	Characteristics and clinical importance
Phosphatidylcholine (Lecithin)	• Present in pulmonary surfactant (Dipalmitoyl lecithin) • Useful in assessment of fetal lung maturity—Amniotic fluid Lecithin/ Sphingomyelin (L/S) ratio • (L/S) ratio ≥2 indicates lung maturity
Sphingomyelin	• Present in surfactant and as the lipid of myelin sheath • Deficiency of the enzyme **sphingomyelinase** leads to **Niemann-Pick disease**
Phosphatidylserine (PS)	• Exposure of PS to the outer surface of cell membrane—an important "eat me" signal for **apoptosis** • Annexin A5 assay is used to detect cells that have expressed PS on the outer cell surface
Phosphatidylinositol (PI)	• Phosphatidylinositol is the precursor of second messenger IP_3 and DAG
Cardiolipin (phosphatidylglycerol)	• Signature phospholipid of mitochondria • The enzyme involved in metabolism of cardiolipin is Tafazzin. Mutation in tafazzin leads to Barth syndrome • Anticardiolipin antibodies are Detected in serodiagnostic flocculation test for syphilis referred to as the Venereal Disease Research Laboratory (VDRL) test

- The glycolipids in cell membrane are **gangliosides and cerebrosides**.
- Glycolipids are particularly abundant in human brain and GIT.
- GM1 Gangliosides act as receptors for the microorganisms infecting human cells like cholera toxin.
- Cell membrane lipids must remain in a state of fluid for optimal functioning.
- Unsaturated fatty acids like linoleic acid, linolenic acid, arachidonic acid, omega-3 fatty acids increase membrane fluidity (Good for Health).
- Saturated fatty acids like stearic acid, palmitic acid decreases membrane fluidity.
- Cholesterol maintains membrane fluidity at an optimal range for proper membrane functioning. That's why cholesterol is also called **Fluidity Buffer.**

Membrane Proteins (Mosaic Component)

Three types of Membrane proteins: Integral membrane proteins, Peripheral membrane proteins and Lipid anchored proteins.

Membrane proteins and their characteristics and clinical importance

Membrane proteins	Characteristics and clinical importance
Integral membrane proteins	• Also called Transmembrane proteins • Functions as receptors (G protein-coupled receptors), channel proteins (Na-K pump), ion channels • CFTR is a transmembrane protein. It is a chloride ion channel. • CFTR mutation—Cystic Fibrosis
Peripheral membrane proteins	• Peripheral proteins are mainly supportive and gives structural integrity • Present in RBC and skeletal muscles • RBC—Spectrin and Ankyrin • Spectrin mutation—Hereditary elliptocytosis • Ankyrin mutation—Hereditary spherocytosis • Skeletal Muscle—Dystrophin • Dystrophin mutation—Duchenne muscular dystrophy • In **Becker muscular dystrophy**, a related disorder, dystrophin is present but altered or reduced in the amount
Lipid anchored proteins	• Also called GPI-anchored proteins • Two GPI-anchored proteins of RBCs namely, CD55 (decay accelerating factor) and CD59 prevents RBCs from hemolysis. • Lack of CD55 and CD59 leads to **Paroxysmal Nocturnal Hemoglobinuria (PNH)**

ENDOPLASMIC RETICULUM

Two types of Endoplasmic reticulum: Rough endoplasmic reticulum (RER) and Smooth endoplasmic reticulum (SER).

Rough Endoplasmic Reticulum (RER)

- Also called granular endoplasmic reticulum because its surface is studded with ribosomes.
- Involved in synthesis of proteins.
- Folding of proteins by chaperones.
- If not properly folded, such as misfolded proteins are degraded by endoplasmic reticulum itself. This function is called Endoplasmic Reticulum Associated Degradation (ERAD).
- Misfolded protein aggregates if not degraded can cause prion disease (PrP^{sc} plaques), Alzheimer's Disease (Aβ Amyloid plaques).

Smooth Endoplasmic Reticulum (SER)

- Also called agranular endoplasmic reticulum because of absence of ribosomes.
- Important for steroid hormone synthesis, storage of calcium in muscle and drug detoxification in liver.

GOLGI APPARATUS

- Mainly involved in sorting of proteins and post-translational processing of proteins.

- The Golgi apparatus is a polarized structure, with cis and trans sides. Cis end is the receiving end. Once processed, the vesicles are released in the form of exocytosis from trans end.
- If Golgi apparatus adds Mannose 6-phosphate to a protein, it will be delivered to lysosomes.
- The enzyme of Golgi apparatus which adds Mannose 6-phosphate is called phosphotransferase. Deficiency of phosphotransferase leads to a disease called **I-cell disease.**

LYSOSOMES

- Cell's digestive organelles (Residual Bodies).
- Highly acidic structures.
- Lysosomal enzymes can hydrolyse virtually every type of biological macromolecule.
- Lysosomes are also called "suicidal bags of the cell", because the interior of lysosomes are always acidic. In the process of destroying the substrate, lysosomes are destroyed along with them.
- Lysosomes are involved in AUTOPHAGY which is a self-destructive process which is activated during starvation to provide energy.

PEROXISOMES (MICROBODIES)

- Involved in generation and degradation of hydrogen peroxide (H_2O_2).
- The defining characteristic of a peroxisome is the presence of **catalase**, an enzyme essential for the degradation of hydrogen peroxide.
- Peroxisomes are involved in oxidation of very long chain fatty acids.
- Peroxisomes are involved in detoxification of harmful chemicals.

MUST KNOW

- Peroxisome biogenesis involves proteins namely peroxins. The gene that encodes peroxin is PEX family of genes. Mutation of these genes leads to **Zellweger syndrome.**
- **Refsum disease:** Autosomal recessive condition due to mutation in gene that encodes for phytanoyl-CoA 2-hydroxylase (PAHX) and peroxin 7 receptor protein (PEX 7)
- **Adrenoleukodystrophy (ALD)** results from a defect in a membrane protein that transports very long chain fatty acids (VLCFA) into the peroxisomes.

MITOCHONDRIA

- Also called "powerhouse of the cell"—involved in the synthesis of ATP by oxidative phosphorylation.
- Mitochondria are derived from the **ovum**, their inheritance is **maternal.**

MUST KNOW

- Human mitochondrial DNA is a double-stranded circular molecule contains approximately 16,500 base pairs
- Large numbers of human diseases are due to mutations in mitochondrial DNA. Muscle and heart are the most affected.
- **MELAS**—Mitochondrial encephalomyopathy, lactic acidosis, and stroke-like episodes; may manifest only as diabetes.

NUCLEUS

- Controls all activities in the cell
- The blue prints—chromosomes
- DNA + Histones = Chromatin
- Chromatin contains repeating structural unit called **nucleosomes**
- Substances can move back and forth nucleus through **nuclear pore complex**
- Proteins of nuclear pore complex—exportins for export and importins for import

MARKER ENZYMES

Certain enzymes are present in certain organelles only. Such specific enzymes are called marker enzymes for that organelle.

Organelle	Marker enzyme
Mitochondria	• Outer membrane—Monoamine oxidase • Inner membrane —ATP synthase, succinate dehydrogenase
Lysosome	• Acid phosphatase
Peroxisomes	• Catalase, urate oxidase
Endoplasmic reticulum	• Glucose-6-phosphatase

Contd...

Organelle	Marker enzyme
Golgi apparatus	• Galactosyltrasferase, Sialyltransferase
Plasma membrane	• 5'-Nucleotidase, $Na^+ K^+$-ATPase
Cytoplasm	• Lactate dehydrogenase

CYTOSKELETAL FILAMENTS

- Play a role in providing strength, support, and cell locomotion.
- Three types of cytoskeletal filaments: Microtubules (largest), Intermediate filaments, Microfilaments (smallest).

1. Microtubules

- Include kinesin, dynein and tubulin
- Help in axonal transport—Dynein—involved in Retrograde (or) reverse axonal transport and Kinesin—involved in Anterograde (or) forward axonal transport
- Dynein helps in movement of cilia, flagella, sperm, fallopian tube
- Cilia helps in clearing sputum from airways
- Cilia is responsible for rotation of internal organs during development
- If Dynein is absent—**Kartagener syndrome** characterized by recurrent sinusitis, male infertility, situs invertus, asthenospermia (Reduced sperm motility)
- **Microtubule-organizing centers (MTOCs)** contain γ-tubulin—helps in movement of chromosomes during cell division
- Microtubule inhibitor drugs—**vincristine, paclitaxel, colchicine**

2. Microfilaments

- Mainly actin and myosin concerned with muscle contraction and cell motility
- **Listeria monocytogenes**—induces actin polymerization- propelled like a rocket (Tumbling Motility) through the cytoplasm of an infected cell

3. Intermediate Filaments

- They are the most abundant cytoskeletal filaments in cell
- Structural proteins of cell which maintains cellular architecture
- Serves as tumor markers

Location and clinical importance of intermediate filaments

Intermediate filaments	Location	Clinical importance
Keratin	Epithelial cells	• Tumor marker -squamous cell carcinoma • Accumulation of keratin in hepatocytes of patients with alcoholic hepatitis is called Mallory—Denk bodies
Desmin	Muscle	• Tumor marker—sarcomas
Vimentin	Mesenchyme	• Tumor marker—melanoma, mesothelioma
Glial Fibrillary Acidic Protein (GFAP)	Astrocytes	• Tumor marker—astrocytoma
Lamin	Nuclear lamina	• Mutation in lamin gene leads to progeria (premature ageing • Progeria syndromes—Werner syndrome ("Progeria of Adult"), Hutchinson-Gilford syndrome ("Progeria of Childhood")

CELL JUNCTIONS

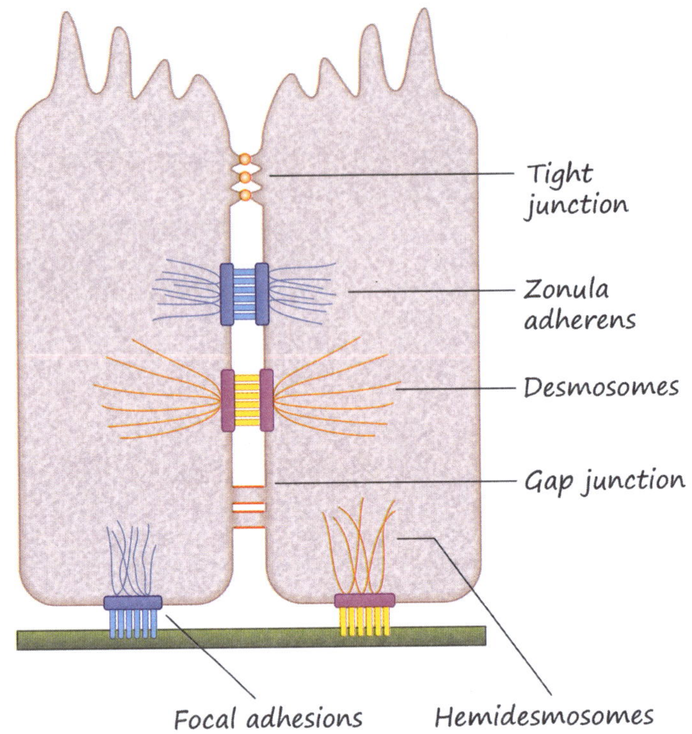

Cell junctions	Characteristics and clinical importance
Zonula adherens	• Linked to the actin cytoskeleton • Primary protein is **E-cadherin** • Listeria monocytogenes contains Internalin A that recognizes E-cadherin (molecular hijacking) and invade the cell
Desmosomes	• Linked to the intermediate filaments • Present in tissues that are subjected to mechanical stress—cardiac muscle skin and uterine cervix • The cadherins of desmosomes—desmogleins and desmocollins • Antibodies against desmogleins—autoimmune disease pemphigus vulgaris
Tight junctions	• Also called **Zonula occludens (ZO)** • Major tight junction proteins—**claudins and occludins** • Tight junctions present in Blood-Brain Barrier • Controls **paracellular** flux of substances between adjacent cells • Mutation in claudin—familial hypomagnesemia with hypercalciuria and nephrocalcinosis
Gap Junctions	• Gap junctions permit substances to pass between the cells without entering the extracellular fluid (ECF) • Gap junction protein—**connexins** • Gap junctions are abundant in **cardiac muscles (intercalated discs)**. It is because of this, cardiac muscle functions as single unit called **functional syncytium** • Gap junctions are also seen in single-unit smooth muscles • Mutations in connexin 40—idiopathic atrial fibrillation • Mutations in connexin 32—X-linked Charcot-Marie-Tooth disease

Contd...

Cell junctions	Characteristics and clinical importance
Hemidesmosomes and focal adhesions	• Mainly connect cell to its basal lamina • Hemidesmosomes are associated with intermediate filaments • Hemidesmosomes contains integrins rather than cadherins • Focal adhesions are associated with actin and are involved in cell movement

CELLULAR RECEPTORS

Cellular receptors are located either in cell membrane (extracellular) or in cytoplasm, nucleus (intracellular).

Cell Membrane Receptors (Extracellular)

Proteins and peptide hormones act through cell membrane receptors

> Cell membrane receptors are of four types. They are:
> 1. G-protein-coupled receptors (GPCRs)
> 2. Receptor tyrosine kinases
> 3. Cytokine receptor family
> 4. Receptor serine/threonine kinase

1. G-protein-coupled receptors (GPCRs)
   - Span the cell membrane seven times. They are also called seven-helix receptors or serpentine receptors
   - Composed of three subunits namely α, β, and γ
   - Once the hormone binds—α-subunit is separated from βγ
   - Energy is provided by hydrolysis of GTP
   - Hormones acting through GPCR are the FIRST MESSENGERS. Inside the cells, downstream actions are mediated through SECOND MESSENGERS

Second messengers		
cAMP	Calcium	cGMP
Hormones causing Water reabsorption, Metabolism, Electrolyte secretion	Hormones causing Contraction, Contraction, Exocytosis	Hormones causing Contraction, Dilatation
Vasopressin (V2) Water reabsorption	Vasopressin (V1) Vasoconstriction	Nitric oxide Vasodilation
Epinephrine (beta) Glycogenolysis	Oxytocin Uterine contraction	Natriuretic peptides Mesangial cell relaxation
Secretin Pancreatic juice rich in bicarbonate	TRH Exocytosis of TSH	

2. Receptor tyrosine kinase—For Insulin
3. Cytokine receptor family Janus kinases (JAK)—for growth hormone, prolactin, leptin, erythropoietin
4. Serine/threonine kinase receptors—for activin, anti-mullerian hormone (AMH)

Nuclear Receptors (Intracellular)

- Unactivated nuclear receptor resides in the cytoplasm for steroid hormones
- Once the hormone binds to the cytoplasmic receptor, the hormone receptor complex moves to the nucleus for all actions
- The receptors located in cytoplasm in inactive state for steroid hormones like:
  - Glucocorticoid receptor
  - Mineralocorticoid receptor
  - Androgen receptor
  - Vitamin D receptor
- Hormones that act through nuclear receptors are:
  - Estrogen Receptor
  - Vitamin A—retinoic acid receptor (RAR)
  - Progesterone receptor
  - Thyroid hormones

MEMBRANE TRANSPORT

Classified as Passive (no need of ATP) and Active transport processes (ATP needed)

Passive Transport

- **Passive processes:** Simple diffusion, facilitated diffusion, osmosis.
- **Simple diffusion:**
  - Diffusion means movement of molecules from area of high concentration to area of low concentration
  - Example: Diffusion of oxygen and carbon dioxide across respiratory membrane. This process is studied using **diffusing capacity of the lungs for carbon monoxide (DLCO)**
  - The law which explains diffusion is called FICK'S LAW

    Fick's Law

    $$\text{Rate of diffusion} = \frac{\text{Membrane surface area} \times \text{conc. gradient}}{\text{Thickness of membrane}}$$
  - Diffusion is directly related to lipid solubility of the substance and inversely related to size of the substance
- **Facilitated diffusion:**
  - Here, the simple diffusion process is facilitated by a carrier protein
  - Example: Glucose transport using GLUT and water transport using aquaporins (AQPs)
  - GLUT4-**Insulin regulated glucose transporter**-Present in Skeletal muscle, heart, adipose tissue
  - Autoantibodies against AQP4 lead to autoimmune demyelinating disease Neuro Myelitis optica (NMO or Devic's syndrome)
- **Osmosis:**
  - Osmosis means DIFFUSION OF WATER. Water moves from area of its high concentration (low solute content) to area of its low concentration (high solute content)
  - One osmole (Osm) corresponds to the number of osmotically active particles
  - **Osmolarity** is the number of osmoles per liter of solution e.g., plasma
  - **Osmolality** is the number of osmoles per kilogram of solvent

> Osmolarity (mOsm/L) = 2 [Na^+] (mEq/L) + 0.055 [Glucose] (mg/dL) + 0.36 [BUN] (mg/dL)
> BUN-Blood Urea Nitrogen
>
> In health, plasma osmolality ranges from 280 mOsm/kg of H_2O to 295 mOsm/kg of H_2O

Active Transport

Classified as Primary active transport and Secondary active transport.

Primary Active Transport

- In primary active transport, the energy is derived directly from breakdown of ATP
- Examples—**Na^+ K^+ ATPase, H^+ K^+ ATPase, Ca^{2+} ATPase**
- Sodium Potassium ATPase:
  - Na-K pump uses the energy to move 3 sodium ions from inside to outside of the cell and moves 2 potassium ions from outside to inside of the cell.
  - The coupling ratio is 3:2
  - It has 2 subunits and both the subunits are different. That is why it is called a heterodimer. The two subunits are α and β
  - The intracellular portion of the α subunit has a Na^+-binding site, a phosphorylation site, and an ATP-binding site
  - The extracellular portion has a K^+-binding site and an ouabain-binding site
  - The β subunit is a glycoprotein which has three extracellular glycosylation sites
  - **Thyroid Hormones, Aldosterone and insulin** increase Na-K pump activity
  - **Dopamine** in the kidney **inhibits** Na-K pump

Secondary Active Transport

- This transport utilizes the energy gradient established by Sodium Potassium ATPase. Here, active transport of sodium is coupled to the transport of other substances
- They can be **cotransporters** where direction of ion movement is the **same** and **antiport or exchangers** where direction of ion movement is **opposite**
- Sodium-Glucose Cotransporter (SGLT)—SGLT 1-intestine, SGLT 2-proximal convoluted tubule of kidney
  - SGLT-1 in intestine is the physiological basis for use of oral rehydration solution (ORS) in diarrheal disorders
  - Congenital absence of SGLT-1 leads to **congenital glucose-galactose malabsorption (CGGM)**
  - Inhibitors of SGLT-2 namely canagliflozin-used in treatment of diabetes mellitus
  - Other examples—sodium iodide cotransporter (NIS), Na^+-K^+-$2Cl^-$ cotransporter (NKCC), chloride bicarbonate exchanger

- Vesicular transport:
  - Classified into two as—Exocytosis (cellular contents are moved out of the cell) and Endocytosis (transport substances from outside to inside of the cell)
    1. **Exocytosis:**
       - The proteins involved in exocytosis are called **SNARE proteins**
       - **Calcium** is required for the process
       - C. botulinum inhibits the release of **acetylcholine** by cleaving the SNARE protein synaptobrevin involved in its exocytosis
       - Since botulinum toxin inhibits the release of acetylcholine, it is useful in conditions characterized by excessive muscle contraction like **Achalasia cardia**
    2. **Endocytosis:**
       - Proteins involved in endocytosis are **clathrin, cubilin and caveolin**
       - Clathrin is required for the endocytosis of LDL receptor cholesterol, transferrin bound iron, nerve growth factor (neurotrophins), hormones (insulin), epidermal growth factor
       - Cubulin—endocytic receptor for intrinsic factor-vitamin B_{12} highly expressed in illeal enterocytes
       - Caveolin is mainly involved in the endocytosis of folate receptor

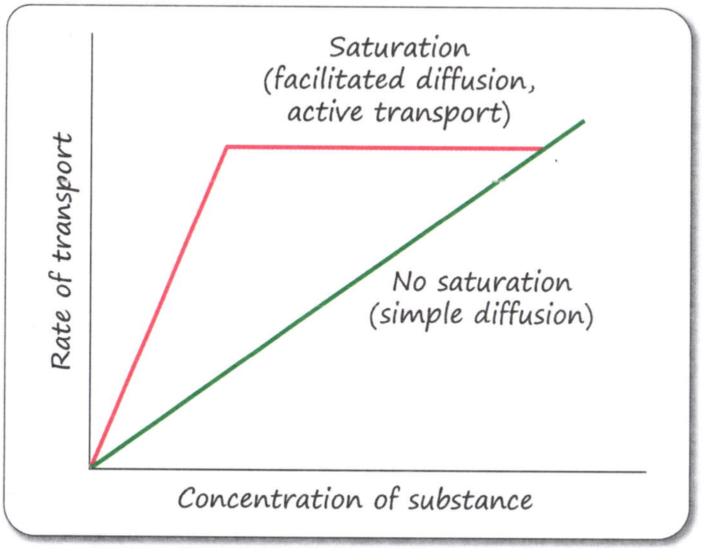

MEMBRANE POTENTIALS

Resting Membrane Potential (RMP)

- At rest, the inside of the cell is negative compared to the exterior. This inside negativity is called resting membrane potential (RMP)
- Passive diffusion of potassium ions from inside to outside of the cell generates RMP

Cell	RMP
Neuron	-70 mV
Skeletal muscle	-90 mV
Cardiac ventricle	-90 mV
Retinal Rods	-40 mV
Inner ear hair cells	-60 mV
Sinoatrial Node	-60 to -40 mV
Gastrointestinal smooth muscle	-60 to -40 mV

Equilibrium Potential

- At a particular membrane potential, an ion cannot move inside the cell and it cannot move outside of the cell too. The membrane potential at which this equilibrium exists is the **equilibrium potential**
- Equilibrium potential for a single ion can be calculated from **Nernst equation**
- Nernst equation: E = ±61 log [X o]/[X i] where E = equilibrium potential, [X o] = concentration outside the cell, [X i] = concentration inside the cell
- Equilibrium potential for multiple ions can be calculated from **Goldman equation**

Ion	Equilibrium potential
Na^+	+60 mV
K^+	-90 mV
Cl^-	-70 mV

Gibbs-Donnan effect

- This effect states that "presence of nondiffusible ions on the one side of cells affects the distribution of permeant (diffusible) ions"
- Nondiffusible anions responsible for the Gibbs-Donnan effect are **protein anions**

CELLULAR FLUIDS

- In a 70-kilogram adult man, maximum percentage contribution (60%) of body weight is WATER.

Total body water divisions between intracellular and extracellular fluid

MUST KNOW

Total body water (60% of body weight), 42 liters		
Intracellular fluid	Extracellular fluid	
2/3rd of TBW i.e., 40% body weight (28 liters)	1/3rd of TBW, i.e., 20% body weight (14 liters)	
	Interstitial fluid	Plasma
	75% or 3/4th of ECF or 15% of body weight (10.5 liters)	25% or 1/4th of ECF or 5% of body weight (3.5 liters)

- The principle employed for **measurement of body fluid volumes** is called **indicator dilution principle.**

Volume	Indicators
Total body water	Deuterium (most used), Tritium, Antipyrine
Extracellular fluid	Inulin (gold standard substance), sucrose, mannitol, sodium thiosulphate
Plasma volume	Evans blue dye, ^{125}I-albumin
Blood volume	^{51}Cr-labeled red blood cells, or calculated as blood volume = plasma volume/(1 - hematocrit)
Interstitial fluid	Calculated as extracellular fluid volume—plasma volume
Intracellular fluid	Calculated as total body water—extracellular fluid volume

- **TOTAL BODY WATER** is more in children (75%) compared to adults (60%).
- Body fat and body water are inversely related.
- Total body water is more in men compared to women.
- **Transcellular Fluids**- subtype of extracellular fluid whose primary function is always lubrication.
- Examples of transcellular fluid are CSF, synovial fluid, pleural fluid, pericardial fluid and aqueous humor.

Compartment	Major cation	Major anion
ECF	Sodium (Na^+)	Chloride (Cl^-)
ICF	Potassium (K^+)	Phosphates (Po_4^{2-})

- **Darrow Yannet Diagram:** Useful to study shifts of water between ECF and ICF compartment.

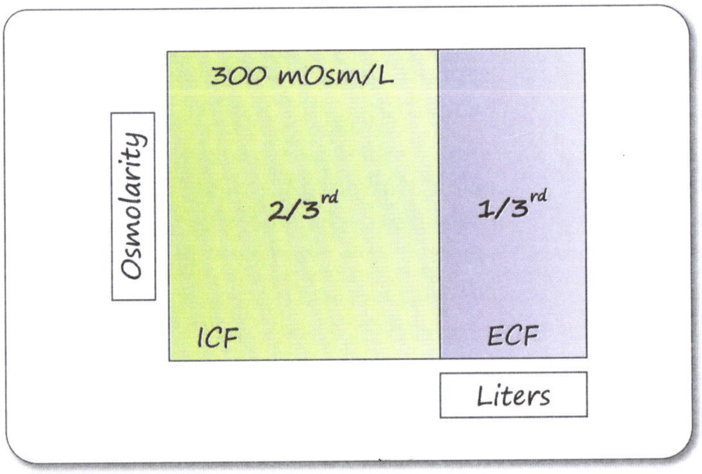

Darrow Yannet Diagram

Excessive intake of NaCl—Hypertension

- The osmolarity of ECF increases because osmoles (NaCl) have been added to the ECF

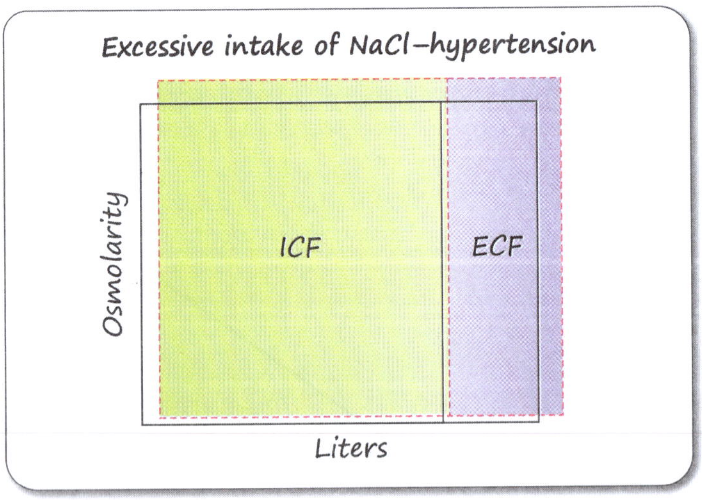

- Water shifts from ICF to ECF. As a result of this shift, **ICF osmolarity increases** until it equals that of ECF.
- As a result of the shift of water out of the cells, **ECF volume increases** and **ICF volume decreases.**

3. NERVE MUSCLE PHYSIOLOGY

STRUCTURE OF A NEURON

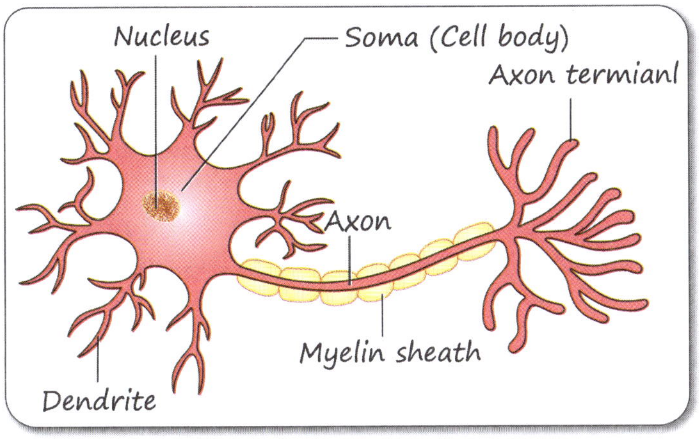

PARTS OF A NEURON ALONG WITH THEIR CHARACTERISTICS

Parts of a neuron	Characteristics
Cell body	• Contains nucleus • Metabolic center
Nissl bodies	• Rough endoplasmic reticulum of neurons
Dendrites	• Receive information • Has small knobby projections called **dendritic spines**
Axon hillock	• Thickened area of the cell body
Axon	• Transmits propagated impulses to the nerve endings
Initial segment	• Site where propagated action potentials are generated
Nerve endings	• Site where neurotransmitters are stored and released

CLASSIFICATION OF NEURONS ALONG WITH THEIR CHARACTERISTICS

Neuron type	Characteristics
Unipolar neurons	• Have a single process originating from the cell body. • Example: Invertebrate neurons

Contd...

Neuron type	Characteristics
Bipolar neurons	• Have two types of processes that are functionally specialized- dendrite and axon. • Examples: Bipolar retinal neurons, olfactory neurons
Pseudo unipolar neurons	• Are variants of bipolar cells in which one end goes to the spinal cord and the other end goes to peripheral skin • Example: Dorsal root ganglion cell
Multipolar neurons	• Have single axon and many dendrites • These are the most common types of neurons in CNS • Examples: Spinal motor neuron, Purkinje cells of cerebellum, sympathetic ganglia

MYELIN

- Myelin insulates nerve fibers and fastens conduction of impulses.
- Myelin speeds impulse conduction by permitting action potentials to jump between naked regions of axons called nodes of Ranvier. Such a type of nerve conduction is called **Saltatory conduction.**
- Myelin is a lipid protein complex. Lipid component is Sphingomyelin; and protein components are Myelin Basic Protein (MBP) and Myelin Oligodendrocyte Glycoprotein (MOG). Autoantibodies are directed against these proteins in a demyelinating disorder called **multiple sclerosis.**
- Myelin is formed by oligodendrocytes in central nervous system and Schwann cells in the peripheral nervous system.
- Oligodendrocyte can myelinate multiple neurons at a time but Schwann cell can myelinate only one neuron at a time.
- **Luxol fast blue:** Special stain for staining myelin sheath.

NERVE ACTION POTENTIAL

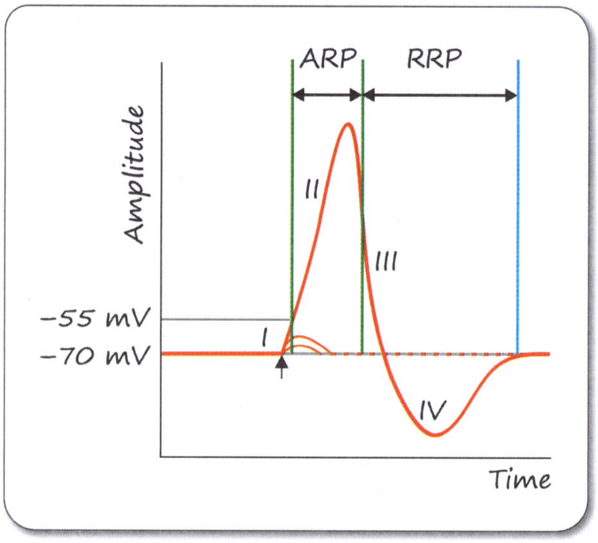

- Phase I: Local potential (–70 mV to –55 mV). Due to slow sodium influx
- Phase II: Depolarization–Rapid sodium influx through voltage gated sodium channels
- Phase III: Repolarization–Potassium efflux
- Phase IV: Hyperpolarization–Delayed closure of potassium channels and also due to chloride influx
- Absolute refractory period (ARP): from firing level (–55 mV) until repolarization is about one-third complete. No stimulus, no matter how strong, will not excite the nerve due to inactivation of sodium channels
- Relative refractory period (RRP): Begins from the remaining part of repolarization to the end of action potential. Stronger than normal stimulus (suprathreshold stimulus) produces action potential

CLASSIFICATION OF NERVE FIBERS

Erlanger and Gasser Classification

Fiber type	Myelin present or absent	Diameter (μm)	Conduction velocity (m/s)	Functions
A α	Myelinated	12-20 (**Largest**)	70–120 (**Highest**)	Proprioception; somatic motor
A β	Myelinated	5-12	30–70	Touch, pressure
A γ	Myelinated	3–6	15–30	Motor to muscle spindles
A δ	Myelinated	2–5	12–30	Pain, temperature
B	Myelinated	<3	3–15	Preganglionic autonomic
C, dorsal root	Unmyelinated	0.4–1.2 (**Smallest**)	0.5–2 (**lowest**)	Pain, temperature
C, Sympathetic	Unmyelinated	0.3–1.3	0.7–2.3	Postganglionic sympathetic

Lloyd Classification

Number	Origin	Fiber type
Ia	Muscle spindle, annulo spiral ending	A α
Ib	Golgi tendon organ	A α
II	Muscle spindle, flower spray ending, touch pressure	A β
III	Pain and cold receptors	A δ
IV	Pain and temperature receptors	C

NERVE INJURY

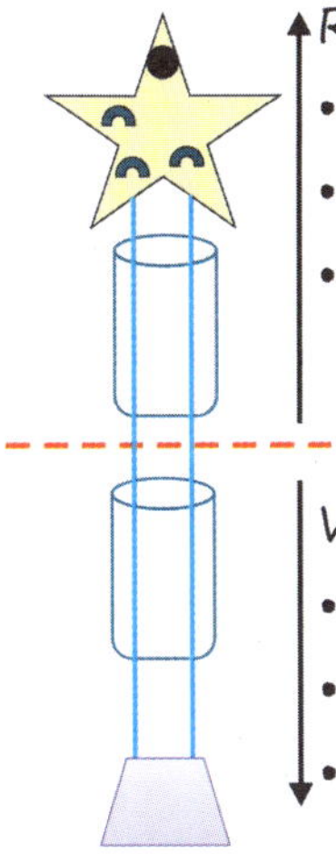

Retrograde (or) proximal degeneration:

- Withing 48 hours of injury and continues up to 15-20 days
- Nucleus is usually pushed toward the periphery
- Rough endoplasmic reticulum of neurons is called Nissl bodies. They undergo degeneration and dissolution. This phenomenon is called chromatolysis

Axonal injury

Wallerian (or) distal degeneration:

- Occurs distal to the site of injury
- Usually begins within 24-36 hours after injury
- Axonal degeneration is the earliest to occur followed by degeneration of myelin sheath
- Macrophages and Schwann cell clear the debris following degeneration

Nerve regeneration:

- With 96 hours of the injury
- Nerve regeneration occurs at the rate of 1-3 mm/day
- **Tinel Sign:** It is done by tapping distal to proximal along the injured nerve. positive sign means it produces **tingling sensation** along the course of the nerve. It is indicative of **nerve regeneration.**

Sunderland Classification with its Equivalent Seddon Classification Terminology and Features

Sunderland classification	Equivalent Seddon classification terminology	Features
First degree	Neuropraxia	• Nerve in continuity • Due to compression or ischemia • Only local conduction block seen • Spontaneous recovery in minutes
Second degree	Axonotmesis	• Injury to axon • Encapsulating structures intact • Wallerian degeneration occurs • Recovery at 1-3 mm/day
Third degree	Neurotmesis	• Injury to axon • Endoneurium disrupted, epineurium and perineurium intact • Wallerian degeneration occurs
Fourth degree	Neurotmesis	• Injury to axon • Endoneurium and perineurium disrupted, only epineurium intact • Wallerian degeneration occurs • Requires surgical intervention for recovery
Fifth degree	Neurotmesis	• Injury to axon • Disruption in all encapsulating layers • Wallerian degeneration occurs • Requires surgical intervention for recovery

SKELETAL MUSCLE

Sarcomere (Functional Units)

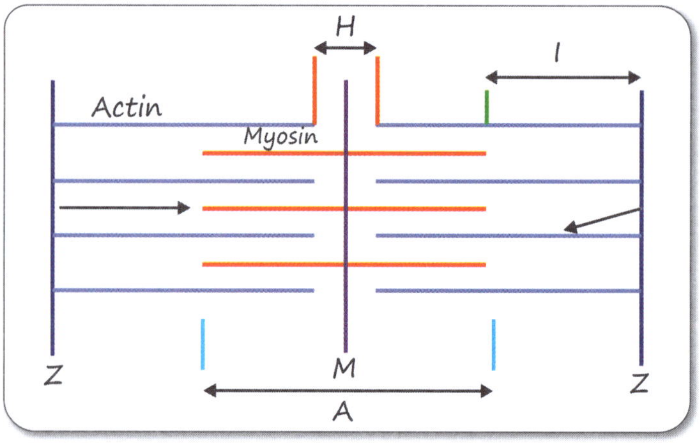

Structure of sarcomere

- Sarcomere—area between two Z lines
- I band—actin filaments (Thin filaments)
- A band—mainly myosin (Thick filaments)
- M line—runs exactly through center of A band
- H band—nonoverlapping part of myosin
- During muscle contraction—Z lines come closer,. Length of H band and I band decreases, A band length remains constant

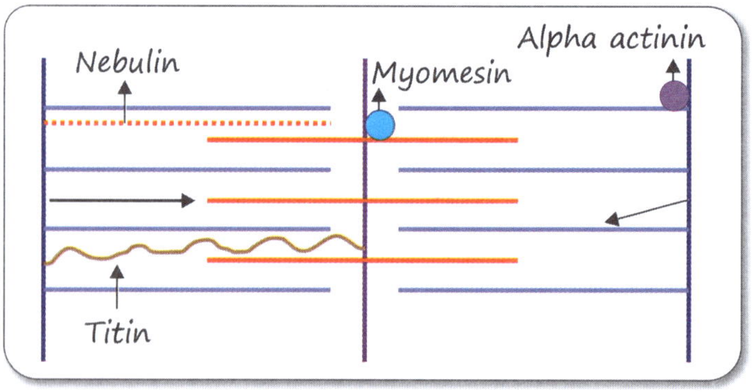

Sarcomere proteins

- Titin
    - Largest known protein present in mammals
    - Muscle spring responsible for "Elasticity"
    - Connects Z line to the M line
- Nebulin
    - Runs along the length of actin
    - Regulates actin length
- Myomesin
    - Attach myosin to M line
- Alpha actinin
    - Attach actin to Z line

Skeletal Muscle Proteins

- **Contractile Proteins:** Actin and Myosin
- **Structural Supporting Proteins:** Titin, Desmin, Dystrophin
- **Regulatory Proteins:** Tropomyosin and Troponin.
    - **Troponin C:** Contains the binding sites for Ca^{2+}.
    - **Troponin I:** Inhibits the interaction of myosin with actin.
    - **Troponin T:** Binds the troponin components to tropomyosin
- **Relaxation Protein: SERCA pump:** Takes up calcium ions leading to muscle relaxation

NEUROMUSCULAR TRANSMISSION AND EXCITATION CONTRACTION COUPLING

- RMP of Neuron is -70 mV

Contd...

- Opening of Voltage gated Na+ channels-Sodium influx leads to RMP change from -70 mV to -40 mV
- Opening of Voltage gated Ca^{2+} channels-Calcium influx
- Exocytosis of Acetylcholine
- Acetylcholine attaches to Nicotinic Ach receptor in Post synaptic end muscle endplate
- Sodium influx into motor endplate—Endplate potential
- Endplate potential summates to produce action potential
- Action potential activates Dihydropyridine Receptor (DHPR)
- DHPR and Ryanodine receptor are mechanically linked and opening of ryanodine receptor leads to calcium release and actin myosin interaction and muscle contraction
- Muscle relaxation is brought about by reuptake of calcium by SERCA pump

Contd...

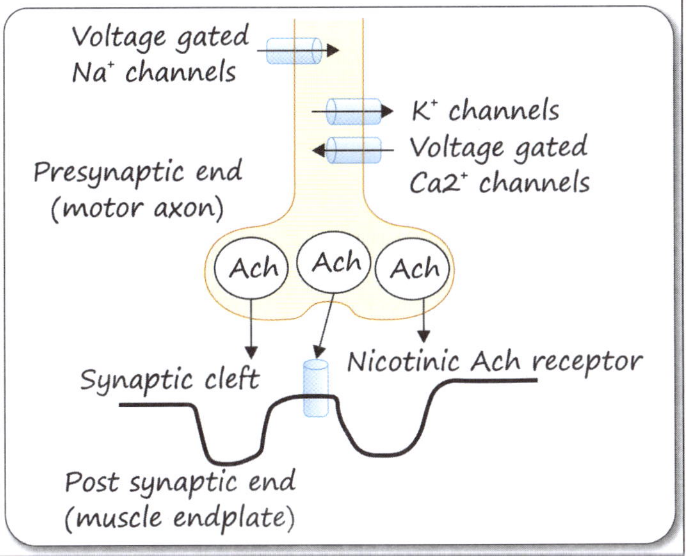

NEUROMUSCULAR BLOCKING AGENTS AND THEIR MECHANISMS OF ACTION

Neuromuscular blocking agent	Mechanism of action
Tetrodotoxin (source—Puffer fish)	Presynaptic voltage-gated sodium channel blocker
Dendrotoxin (source—Mamba snake)	Presynaptic voltage-gated potassium channel blocker
Conotoxin (source—Snail)	Presynaptic voltage-gated calcium channel blocker
Botulinum Toxin	Inhibits release of Acetylcholine leading to flaccid paralysis

NEUROMUSCULAR JUNCTION AND DISEASES

Myasthenia Gravis	Lambert Eaton Myasthenia Syndrome
• Myasthenia gravis (MG) is an autoimmune disease due to auto antibodies directed against nicotinic acetylcholine receptors (AChRs). It is a postsynaptic disorder • The cardinal features are weakness and fatigability of muscles but deep tendon reflexes are preserved • The amount of ACh released per impulse normally declines on repeated activity. It is the reason behind **decremental response** seen in repeated nerve stimulation in myasthenia gravis called **myasthenic fatigue.**	• Lambert Eaton Myasthenia Syndrome (LEMS) is a presynaptic disorder • LEMS is caused by autoantibodies directed against P/Q-type calcium channels at the motor nerve terminals • It is distinguished from myasthenia gravis by two important reasons. One, LEMS have depressed or absent reflexes and two, high frequency repetitive nerve stimulation causes incremental response in LEMS

MUSCLE CONTRACTION: SLIDING FILAMENT THEORY

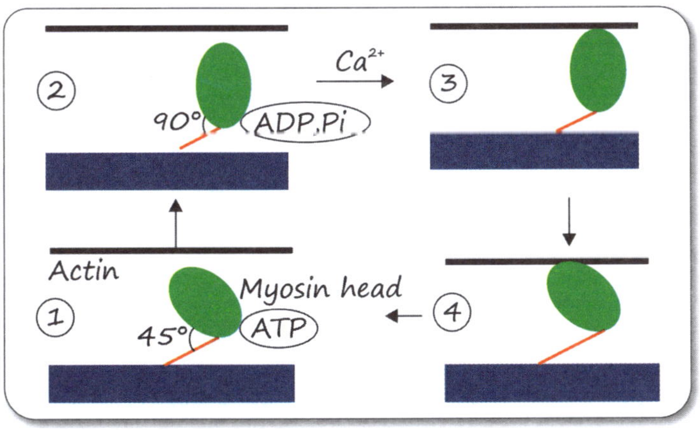

Muscle contraction, sliding filament theory

Step 1

- **Myosin head at 45°** during resting state
- ATP binding to myosin head activates myosin ATPase
- ATP hydrolysis to ADP and Pi

Step 2

- Myosin head moves from 45° to 90°
- Myosin head contains ADP and Pi

Step 3

- In presence of calcium, actin and myosin interacts
- Formation of crossbridge

Step 4

- **ADP and Pi are released from myosin head**
- **Myosin head tilts back to 45°** (Power Stroke)
- Myosin head detachment from actin require a new molecule of ATP attachment to myosin head
- After death—No ATP—No myosin head detachment leads to RIGOR MORTIS (Sustained Contraction)

LENGTH-TENSION RELATIONSHIP: SKELETAL MUSCLE

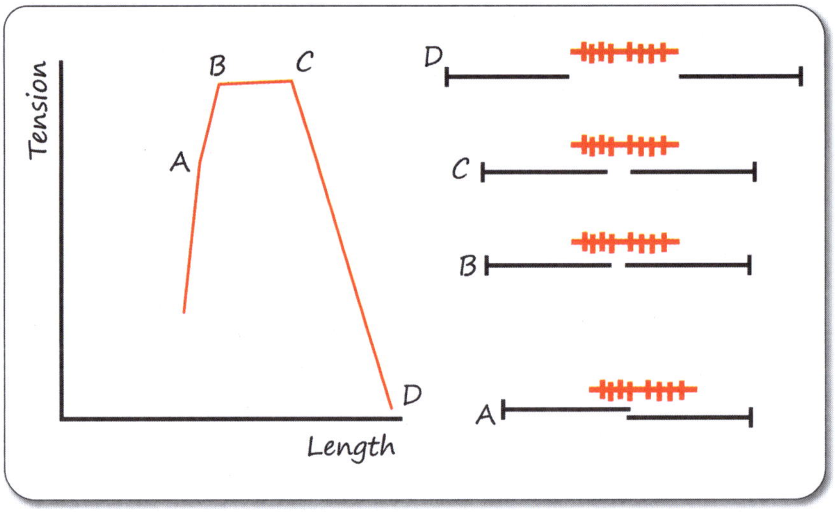

- Maximum tension generated by the muscle is between point B and C
- It corresponds to the sarcomere length of 2.2 micrometers.
- It Is at this segment BC where there is optimal overlap between actin and myosin
- On either side of BC, tension produced by the muscle decreases

SKELETAL MUSCLE FIBER TYPES

Characteristics of Skeletal Muscle Fibers

Characteristics	Type I fibers	Type II fibers	
		Type II a	Type II b
Other names	Slow oxidative	Fast oxidative glycolytic	Fast glycolytic
Myoglobin content	High	High	Low
Color	Red	Red	White
Myosin ATPase activity	Slow	Fast	Fast
Ca^{2+} pumping capacity of SR	Moderate	High	High
Diameter	Small	Large	Large
Glycolytic capacity	Moderate	High	High
Oxidative capacity	High	Moderate	Low
Associated with motor unit type	Slow	Fast resistant to fatigue	Fast fatigable
Recruitment order	First	Second	Third
Activities best suited for	Maintaining posture, Endurance type activities (running a marathon)	Walking	Sprinting
Mitochondria	Many	Many	Few
Capillaries	Many	Many	Few

Motor Unit

- Each single motor neuron and the muscle fibers it innervates constitute a motor unit.
- Motor unit innervates very few (three to six) muscle fibers in muscles concerned with fine, precise, graded movements like extra ocular muscles and hand muscles. In leg muscles, motor unit innervates up to 600 muscle fibers.

Size Principle

- Small diameter slow type I fibers are always recruited first. They are followed by recruitment of Type II a fatigue resistant fiber.
- Last to be recruited are the Type II b fast fatigable fibers.

CARDIAC MUSCLE

- Striated, Involuntary
- Have Intercalated Disk-Cardiac Gap junctions
- **Connexins:** Proteins present in Gap Junction
- **Functional syncytium:** cardiac muscle fibers contract together all at the same time because of the presence of Gap junctions
- **Calcium-induced calcium release (CICR):** Calcium from extracellular source should come first to release calcium from intracellular source in cardiac muscle.

SMOOTH MUSCLE

- Involuntary
- Single unit and Multi unit—Single unit smooth muscle has Gap junctions.
- Single unit smooth muscle is found in visceral organs namely uterus, intestine, ureter and urinary bladder.
- Multi-unit smooth muscle is found in iris, ciliary body, epididymis, vas deferens, piloerector muscle of skin.
- Blood vessels got both single unit and multi-unit smooth muscle in their walls.
- No Z lines—equivalent is Dense bodies
- Calmodulin—Calcium binding protein. No Troponin
- **Plasticity:** If visceral smooth muscle is stretched, it first exerts increased tension. However, if the muscle is held at the greater length after stretching, the tension gradually decreases. This initial increase in tension later followed by decrease is called plasticity.
- **Latch Bridge Mechanism:** Smooth muscle can be maintained in a prolonged state of partial contraction (tonus) with very little use of ATP. This is due to latch bridge mechanism in which myosin cross-bridges remain attached to actin for some time after the cytoplasmic Ca^{2+} concentration falls.
- The type of **neuromuscular junction in smooth muscle** wherein one neuron innervating multiple smooth muscle cells is called **synapse en passant.**

SYNAPTIC POTENTIALS

- Synaptic potentials can be excitatory postsynaptic potentials (EPSPs) or inhibitory post synaptic potentials (IPSPs).
- EPSP and IPSP can be fast or slow.
- **Fast EPSP:** Due to influx of sodium or calcium (cell interior more positive).
- **Fast IPSP:** Due to influx of chloride (cell interior more negative).
- **Slow EPSP:** Due to reduced potassium efflux (cell interior more positive).
- **Slow IPSP:** Due to increase in potassium efflux (cell interior more negative).
- Slow EPSP and IPSP are commonly seen in autonomic ganglia, cardiac and smooth muscles.

INHIBITION AND FACILITATION AT SYNAPSES

- **Postsynaptic inhibition:** Hyperpolarization is caused by the inhibitory neurotransmitters GABA and Glycine on a postsynaptic neuron. Also called **afferent inhibition.**
- **Presynaptic inhibition:** Occurs at the presynaptic terminals before the signal ever reaches the synapse by GABA. Also called **lateral inhibition.**
- **Renshaw cell inhibition:** Renshaw cells are excited by a motor neuron. In turn, Renshaw cells inhibit the same motor neuron which excites it. Neurotransmitter involved is GLYCINE. Also called "negative feedback inhibition".

NEUROTRANSMITTERS

Some of the major neurotransmitters are as follows:

Acetylcholine	• Functions as transmitter at—neuromuscular junction, autonomic ganglia, and in postganglionic parasympathetic, basal forebrain complex, Ponto mesencephalic cholinergic complex • Involved in regulation of sleep-wake states, learning and memory • Receptors: 2 types • **Muscarinic:** (M_1, M_4, and M_5-CNS), (M_2-Heart), (M_3-glands and smooth muscles) • **Nicotinic:** (N_M- neuromuscular junction), (N_N- CNS and autonomic ganglia)
Norepinephrine	• Location- locus coeruleus • Activates reticular activating system • Responsible for Awake arousal state
Dopamine	• Location—Nigrostriatal system (motor movements), mesocortical system (Ventral tegmental area nucleus accumbens for motivation and addiction) and Tuberoinfundibular system (inhibits prolactin) • Involved in addiction, reward • Receptors: D_1, D_2, D_3, D_4, D_5 (All are G Protein Coupled Receptors)
Serotonin	• Present in highest concentration in blood platelets and in the gastrointestinal tract • Also, in midline raphe nuclei • Responsible for Awake arousal state, platelet aggregation, peristalsis
Histamine	• Location—posterior hypothalamus • Responsible for awake arousal state
Glutamate	• Major excitatory neurotransmitter in CNS • Location—Hippocampus, Subthalamic Nuclei • Important for learning and memory
GABA	• Major Inhibitory neurotransmitter • Causes hyperpolarization due to chloride influx leading to inhibition of neuronal functions
Glycine	• Both inhibitory and excitatory neurotransmitter • Found in Renshaw cells in spinal cord • Antagonist—Strychnine
Nitric Oxide	• Gaseous neurotransmitter found in Hippocampus • Role in learning and memory
Carbon Monoxide	• Gaseous neurotransmitter produced by enzymatic degradation of heme by heme oxygenase • Role in learning and memory, pain processing, olfaction

4. NEUROPHYSIOLOGY

- Two types of cells are seen in central nervous system: nerve cells or neurons and glial cells.
- Glial cells are 10 times more in number than neurons.

Types of glial cells are astrocytes, oligodendrocytes, Schwann cells and microglial cells.

- Astrocytes:
  - Seen as two groups—Fibrous astrocytes seen in white matter and Protoplasmic astrocytes seen in gray matter.
  - Astrocytes are involved in the formation of the blood-brain barrier.
  - Astrocytes also take up neurotransmitters and K^+ ions from synapses after release from neurons.
  - Astrocytes produce substances that are the major nourishment for neurons namely neurotrophins
- Oligodendrocytes—myelination neurons in the central nervous system.
- Schwann cell causes myelination of neurons in the peripheral nervous system.
- Microglial cells are phagocytic cells.

SENSORY PHYSIOLOGY

- Classified as somatic senses (touch, pain, temperature) and special senses (vision, hearing, smell, taste, balance).
- Somatic senses are conveyed by receptors in skin through first order neurons to spinal cord (second order neurons), to thalamus (ventroposterolateral nucleus third order neurons) and finally to Somatosensory cortex.

TOUCH RECEPTORS

Touch receptors along with their characteristics are as follows:

Touch receptors	Characteristics
Meissner corpuscles	• Mainly detect the initial contact of the hand with objects • Respond to changes in texture • Respond to low frequency slow vibrations
Merkel cells	• Sensitive to edges, corners and points • Distinguish textures—play key roles in the ability to read Braille for blind people
Pacinian corpuscles	• Detect deep pressure and high frequency fast vibration
Ruffini corpuscles	• Seen around joint capsules • They respond to sustained pressure • They are very sensitive to skin stretch

Contd...

MUST KNOW

- **Meissner corpuscles** and **Pacinian corpuscles** are rapidly adapting receptors.
- **Merkel cells** and **Ruffini corpuscles** are slowly adapting receptors.

PAIN RECEPTORS

- Pain receptors are free nerve endings. They are slowly adapting receptors.
- Pain sensation is carried by Aδ fibers and C fibers.

Aδ fibers	C fibers
• Thinly myelinated • responsible for first pain • This type of pain is also called fast pain or epicritic pain • Mainly responsible for localizing the site and intensity of the noxious stimulus • Relatively new in evolution- carried by neospinothalamic tract • Release glutamate as neurotransmitter	• Unmyelinated • responsible for second pain • This type of pain is also called slow pain, protopathic pain • Always dull, intense, diffuse, and gives unpleasant feeling • Very old in evolution- carried by paleospinothalamic tract • Release substance P as neurotransmitter

Gate Control Theory of Pain

- Proposed by Melzack and Wall.
- In Substantia Gelatinosa of spinal cord.

- Dorsal horn neuron receives collaterals from both the touch receptors and pain receptors. Simultaneous activation of innocuous touch receptors reduces the responsiveness of dorsal horn neurons to their input from pain receptor afferents.
- It is the basis behind transcutaneous electrical nerve stimulation (TENS) wherein electrodes are used to activate Aα and Aβ fibers near the site of injury to relieve pain.
- Also, the reason for massaging and applying counterirritants over the injured area relieves pain.

SOMATOSENSORY PATHWAYS

- Dorsal column pathway—Principal pathways for touch, vibration and proprioception. They primarily contain Aα and Aβ afferents. They ascend ipsilaterally (same side) in dorsal column of spinal cord to medulla. In medulla, they synapse with two important nuclei, namely gracilus and cuneate nuclei.
- Anterolateral spinothalamic tract—Principal pathways for pain and temperature sensation. They cross the midline in spinal cord itself (contralateral tract).
- Brown-Sequard syndrome:
  - Ipsilateral loss of joint position and vibratory sense (dorsal column)
  - Contralateral loss of pain and temperature sense (anterolateral spinothalamic tract)
  - Ipsilateral weakness (corticospinal tract) below the lesion

Thalamus

- Thalamus is the general "sensory relay station".
- Somatic senses reach ventroposterolateral (VPL) nuclei of thalamus.

Somatosensory Cortex

- Primary somatosensory cortex is located in post central gyrus of the parietal lobe, Brodmann area—Areas 3, 1, 2
- Major function of somatosensory cortex is localization of the stimulus.
- Exact localization is possible because all our body regions are represented in the cortex. This representation is called **Homunculus.**

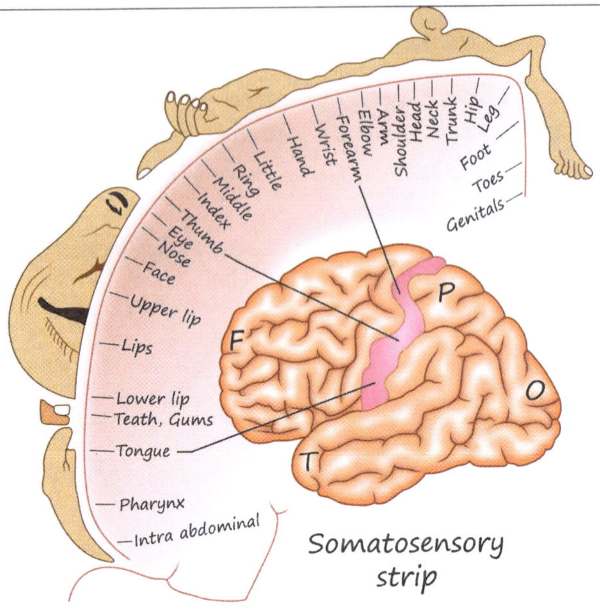

Somatosensory strip

Sensory Homunculus

- Size of the cortical receiving area for impulses from a particular part of the body is proportional to the use of the part.
- Body parts are represented with foot on top most medially and head most laterally.
- Lips and thumb have maximum representation.
- Representations for trunk and back are small.

SPECIAL SENSES

Vision

- Visual information is processed at three important regions, which are retina, lateral geniculate body (thalamus) and visual cortex.
- Retina has seven types of cells.

Retinal cell	Characteristics
Rods	• There are 120 million rods in each human eye. • They are the receptors of dim vision or night vision.
Cones	• There are 6 million cones in each human eye. • They are the receptors of day vision.
Bipolar cells	• They receive signals from rods and cones and make connection with ganglion cells.

Contd...

Retinal cell	Characteristics
Ganglion cells	• They are the only output cell of retina. Their axons are the optic nerve. • They are the only retinal cell capable of producing action potential.
Horizontal cells	• They connect rods and cones. • They sharpen the signal by lateral inhibition.
Amacrine cells	• They are the purely depolarizing cells of retina. • They connect ganglion cells and bipolar cells. • They sharpen the signal by lateral inhibition.
Muller cells	• They are the supporting glial cells. • They have no role in visual processing.

Rods—dark state	Rods—Light state
• cGMP dependent sodium channels (Funny current channels) open leading to depolarization. • Glutamate release happens.	• Light converts 11 cis retinal to All trans retinal which activates transducin. • Transducin activates phosphodiesterase that degrades cGMP and closure of sodium channels • Hyperpolarization • Decrease in glutamate release

Lateral Geniculate Body

- Each lateral geniculate body (LGB) contains six well-defined layers.
- Layers 1 and 2 have large cells—called Magnocellular layer.
- Layers 3, 4, 5 and 6 have small cells—called Parvocellular layer.
- On each side, layers 1, 4 and 6 receive input from the contralateral eye, while layers 2, 3 and 5 receive input from the ipsilateral eye.

Magnocellular pathway versus parvocellular pathway

	Magnocellular pathway	Parvocellular pathway
Origin	Layers 1 and 2 of LGB	Layers 3, 4, 5 and 6 of LGB
Termination	Layer 4 of visual cortex	Layer 4 of visual cortex
Function	Carries signal for detection of movement, depth and flicker	Carries signal for detection of: color vision, texture, shape and fine detail

Visual Cortex

- Visual cortex is located in calcarine sulcus in the occipital lobe; Brodmann areas 17, 18 and 19
- It is heavily myelinated and appears as stripes or stria. It is also called **striate cortex** or stria of Gennari.
- Contains simple cells, complex cells and blobs (Color Vision).
- Color Vision:
    - Cones in retina are the receptors for color vision.
    - Three primary colors are blue, green and red. Correspondingly human retina has three types of cones namely **Blue-sensitive or short wave or S cone, Green-sensitive or middle-wave or M cone and Red-sensitive or long-wave or L cone.**
    - Protanopia (complete red color defect), deuteranopia (complete green color defect) and tritanopia (complete blue color defect).
    - Color Blindness—Transmitted as X-linked recessive. Males are commonly affected. Red green defect is more common.
- Any area other than primary visual cortex which receives visual information is called "Extra striate cortex". They are parietal cortex (concerned with motion or movement of visual stimulus) and temporal cortex (concerned with shape and recognition of faces).

Order of neurons in visual pathway	
Rods and cones (Photoreceptors)	First order neurons
Bipolar cells	Second order neurons
Ganglion cells	Third order neurons
Lateral geniculate body	Fourth order neurons
Visual cortex	Fifth order neurons

Hearing

Human cochlea in the inner ear has receptors for hearing namely hair cells.

Cochlea

- The upper scala vestibuli and the lower scala tympani contain perilymph which is rich in sodium ion
- The scala media is the middle cochlear chamber which has stria vascularis that secretes endolymph which is rich in potassium ion
- Scala media is electrically positive by 85 mV (Endo cochlear potential) relative to the scala vestibuli and scala tympani

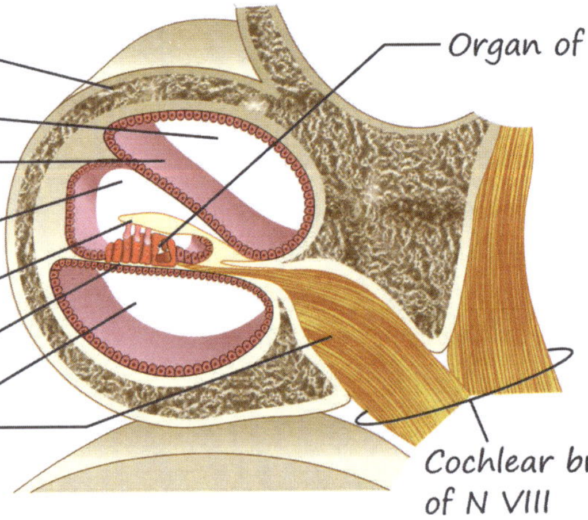

Organ of Corti

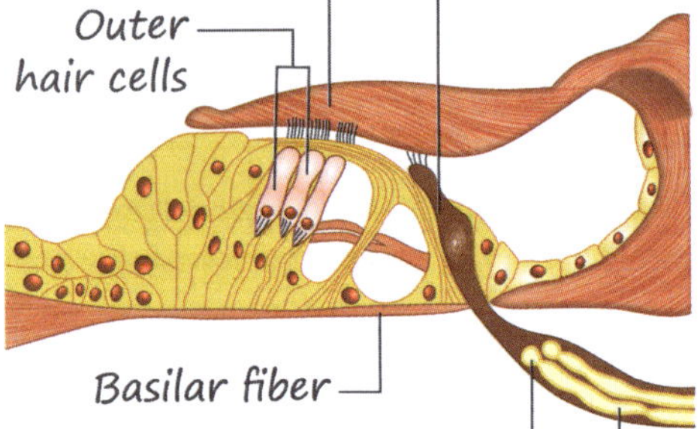

- Contains the receptors for hearing -Hair cells
- Types of hair cells—Outer hair cells and inner hair cells
- 95% of the sensory neurons innervate the inner hair cells; only 5-10% innervate the outer hair cells
- Hair cells have a motor protein namely prestin
- The tallest cilia in hair cel l is called as Kinocilium and the progressively shorter ones are called at Stereocilia
- When the entire hair cells bend towards the tallest one-influx of potassium-depolarization and activation.
- When all the hair cells bend away from the tallest one-inhibition

Role of basilar membrane in hearing process—The frequency analyzer

- Sound waves produce vibrations of the basilar membrane.
- The basilar membrane is thin at the apex of the cochlea but thicker and tauter toward the base.
- **High-frequency sounds** vibrate basilar membrane best near the base of the cochlea, while **low-frequency sounds** vibrate basilar membrane best near the apex of the cochlea—This aspect of basilar membrane gives it the name **The frequency analyzer.**
- This gives the appearance of a **traveling wave** in basilar membrane—This theory is called the **traveling wave theory of von Békésy.**

Central Auditory Pathway

Auditory pathway can be easily remembered with the help of a very familiar mnemonic E COLI MA.

Mnemonic: E COLI MA.

Eighth nerve

Cochlear nuclei

Superior Olivary nucleus

- Helps in localization of sound and the direction from which the sound comes

Lateral lemniscus

Inferior colliculus

- Helps in localization of sound and the direction from which the sound comes

Medial geniculate body—Thalamic nuclei for hearing

Auditory cortex

- Location—superior temporal gyrus of the temporal lobe
- Brodmann area 41
- Also called **Heschl gyrus**
- **Planum temporale:** Part of auditory cortex involved in language-related auditory processing. It is larger in the left hemisphere.

Olfaction (Smell)

- **Olfactory receptors:** Bipolar neurons located in roof of the nasal cavity in a specialized region called **olfactory epithelium.**
- **Basal stem cells:** Source of new olfactory neurons to replace damaged ones
- The Nobel Prize in physiology or medicine 2004 was awarded to Linda Buck and Richard Axel for their discoveries of odorant receptors and organization of olfactory system.
- **Olfactory bulb**
  - Olfactory sensory neurons pass through the cribriform plate of the ethmoid bone and enter the olfactory bulbs
  - Contains four cells; two excitatory cells namely mitral, tufted cells; and two inhibitory cells namely granule cells, periglomerular cells.
- Traditionally, it is stated that olfactory sense bypasses the thalamus.
- A newer pathway is found out in which olfactory signals pass through dorsomedial thalamic nucleus to the orbitofrontal cortex.

Functions of the central areas concerned with olfaction

Central Area	Function
Olfactory cortex—Orbitofrontal cortex	Conscious discrimination of odors
Amygdala	Emotional responses to olfactory stimuli
Entorhinal cortex	Concerned with olfactory memories

Taste (Gustation)

- The specialized sense organ for taste is called taste bud.
- Five basic taste sensations of humans are sweet, salt, sour, bitter and umami.
- Umami is the recently added fifth taste sensation produced by monosodium glutamate (MSG).

Taste	Receptor
Salt	Epithelial Na channels (ENaCs)
Sour	Epithelial Na channels (ENaCs)
Sweet	GPCR T1R2 and T1R3 family receptors
Bitter	GPCR T2R family receptors
Umami	GPCR mGluR4 receptor

Taste Pathways

Taste information from the mouth is carried by three cranial nerves

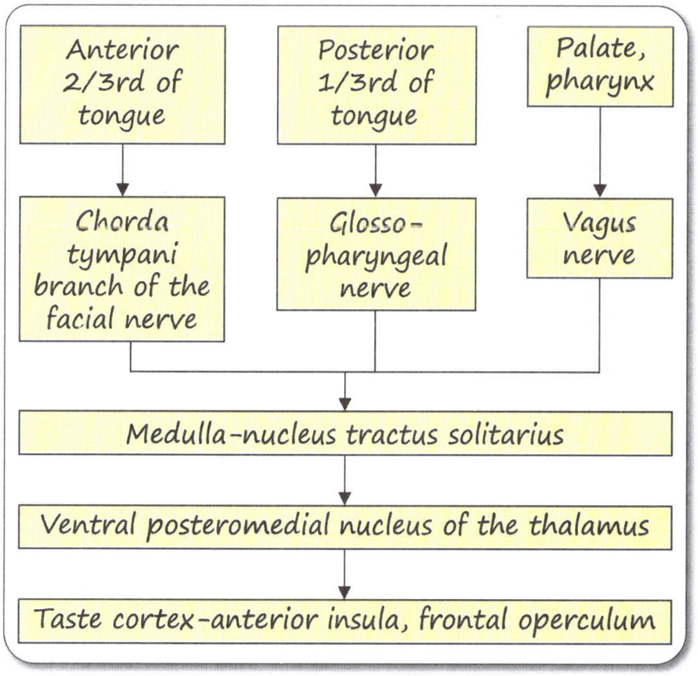

LAWS AND PRINCIPLES IN SENSORY PHYSIOLOGY

- **Doctrine of specific nerve energies (Muller):** Receptors are specialized for a particular sensation. Example: Free nerve endings for pain.
- **Bell-Magendie law:** "Spinal dorsal roots contain sensory fibers and ventral roots contain motor fibers".
- **Law of projection:** Cortex projects sensation to the location of receptor. This law explains phantom pain where patients complain of pain and proprioceptive sensations in the absent limb after amputation.
- **Weber-Fechner law:** "The magnitude of the sensation felt is proportionate to the log of the intensity of the stimulus".

MOTOR PHYSIOLOGY

Terms and their meanings in motor physiology

Term	Meaning
Upper motor neurons	• Cortical and brainstem neurons involved in motor control
Lower motor neurons	• Spinal anterior horn motor neurons • They are the **final common path** for all motor movements
Pyramidal tract	• The other name for corticospinal tract
Extrapyramidal tract	• Any tract other than corticospinal tract that is involved in motor control • Vestibulospinal, reticulospinal, rubrospinal and tectospinal pathways
Lateral motor system	• Mainly the Corticospinal and rubrospinal pathways • Main function—controls fine, skilled voluntary movements involving distal muscles
Medial motor system	• Mainly the vestibulospinal, reticulospinal and tectospinal pathways • Main function—Maintenance of posture that involves proximal muscles

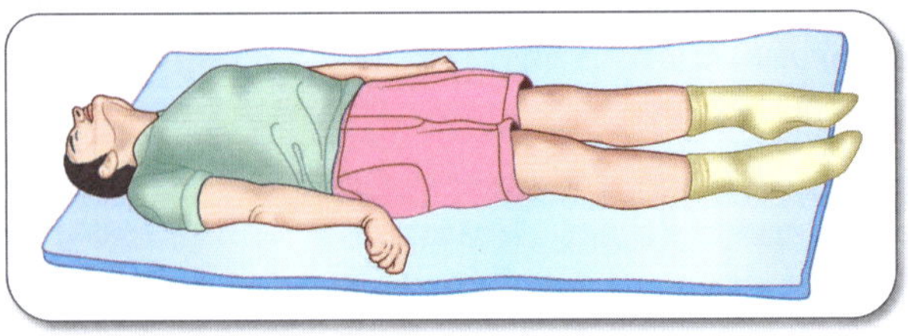

Decerebrate rigidity

Decerebration: A complete transection of the brainstem between the superior and inferior colliculi.

In decerebrate rigidity:

- Lower extremities are extended
- Toes point inward
- Upper extremity is extended
- Fingers flexed and the forearms pronated
- Neck and head are extended

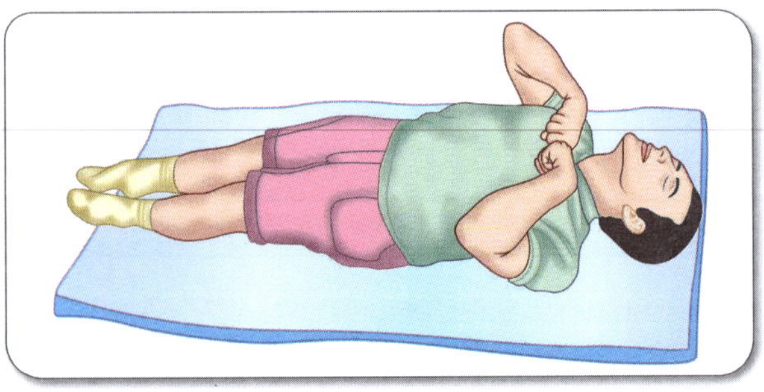

Decorticate rigidity

Decortication:

- Removal of the cerebral cortex
- Influence of corticospinal tract on lower brainstem motor pathways is lost
- **Rubrospinal tract is intact**
- The rubrospinal tract influences primarily **flexor muscles of upper extremity**

  In decorticate rigidity:
  - The lower extremities are extended
  - Toes point slightly inward
  - **Upper extremities are flexed against the chest**
  - The head is extended

REFLEX

Stretch Reflex and Inverse Stretch Reflex

Characteristics of stretch reflex and inverse stretch reflex

Characteristics	Stretch reflex	Inverse stretch reflex
Stimulus	Passive stretch of muscle	Both passive stretch and active contraction
Receptor	Muscle spindle	Golgi tendon organ
Location of receptor	Muscle spindle is parallel to muscle fibers	Golgi tendon organ lies in series to muscle fibers
Detects	Muscle length	Force or tension generated in muscle
Afferent	group Ia endings and group II endings	group Ib endings
Center	Spinal cord	Spinal cord
Efferent	Alpha motor neuron	Alpha motor neuron
Effect	Muscle contraction	Muscle relaxation
Reason for the effect	Alpha motor neuron activated	Alpha motor neuron inhibited
Gamma motor innervation	Present. Innervates the peripheral contractile part of spindles	Absent
Number of synapses involved	Single—Monosynaptic reflex	Two—Disynaptic reflex
Another name of the reflex	Myotatic reflex	Lengthening reaction

The Withdrawal Reflex

- Occurs in response to painful stimulation of the skin or subcutaneous tissues.
- Response—flexor muscle contraction and inhibition of extensor muscles on the affected limb muscle—this is mainly to withdrawn limb away from the stimulus.
- In the opposite limb—extension occurs—this is mainly to support the body.
- The withdrawal reflex-classical example of polysynaptic reflex.

CEREBELLUM

- Cerebellum does start stop signaling. It starts and stops a motor movement. This is needed for proper coordination of motor movements (major function).
- It has three parts, three functions, four deep nuclei and five cells.
- Three parts of cerebellum are Spinocerebellum for coordination function, Vestibulocerebellum for balance and equilibrium and finally Neocerebellum for planning motor movements.
- Four deep Nuclei-Dentate, Emboliform, Fastigial, Globose. All are excitatory.
- Five cells—Purkinje cells, Stellate cells, Golgi cells, Basket cells, Granule cells.
- All the cerebellar cells are inhibitory except Granule cells (excitatory).
- Two main types of afferent fibers that reach the cerebellum are climbing fibers and mossy fibers.
- **Climbing fibers:** Originate in the inferior olivary nucleus (olivocerebellar). **Mossy fibers-** Originate from cell bodies in the spinal cord (Spinocerebellar).
- Climbing fibers directly excite cerebellar deep nuclei initially (START SIGNAL) and later they travel up in cerebellum and excite Purkinje cells.
- Purkinje cells in turn inhibit deep nuclei (STOP SIGNAL). So, there is strong excitation to deep nuclei followed later by inhibition.
- Mossy fiber excites Granule cells.
- Granule cells (parallel fibers) in turn excite stellate, basket and Golgi cells. This is called **feed forward activation.**
- Stellate and basket cells inhibit Purkinje cells. This is called **feed forward inhibition.**
- To regulate granule cell output, Golgi cells inhibit granule cells back. This is called **feedback inhibition.**

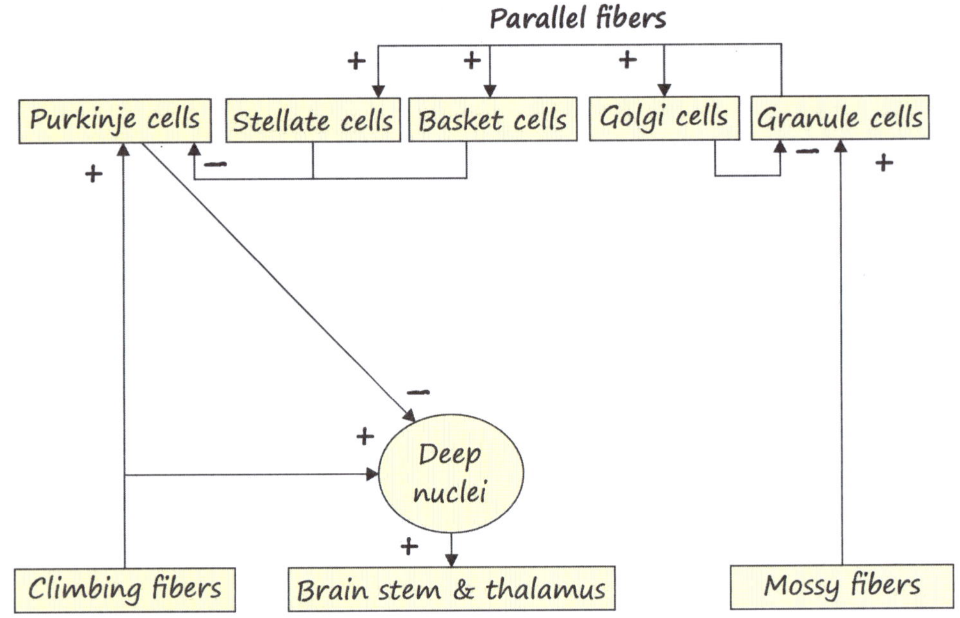

MUST KNOW

Features of cerebellar disease are as follows:

- **Decomposition of movement**
- **Hypotonia:** Decrease in muscle tone
- **Pendular knee jerk**
- **Ataxia:** Leading to unsteady gait
- **Dysmetria:** Also called past-pointing
- **Intention tremor:**
    - Seen when the patient performs a voluntary movement as the endpoint or target is approached
    - This is opposite to that seen in patients with Parkinson's disease, where tremor is evident at rest (**resting tremor**)
- **Dysdiadochokinesia:** Inability to perform rapidly alternating opposite movements such as repeated pronation and supination of the hands
- **Rebound phenomenon**
- **Dysarthria**
- **Scanning speech**
- **Nystagmus**

BASAL GANGLIA

- Basal ganglia suppress both voluntary and involuntary motor movements. At rest, basal ganglia output is inhibitory.
- Components of basal ganglia are Caudate, Putamen, Globus pallidus, Substantia nigra and Subthalamic nucleus.
- Caudate and Putamen-Collectively called striatum—major input nuclei-neurotransmitter GABA. Caudate nucleus plays a role in cognition (learning and memory).
- Globus pallidus has two segments: external and internal segments (GPe and GPi). GPi is the major output nuclei of basal ganglia- neurotransmitter GABA. Tonically active at rest. This is the reason why output of basal ganglia is inhibitory at rest.
- The substantia nigra is divided into Pars compacta, which uses dopamine as a neurotransmitter and Pars reticulata, which uses GABA as a neurotransmitter.
- Subthalamic nucleus—also called Luys' body. Contains the excitatory neurotransmitter Glutamate

Direct Pathway

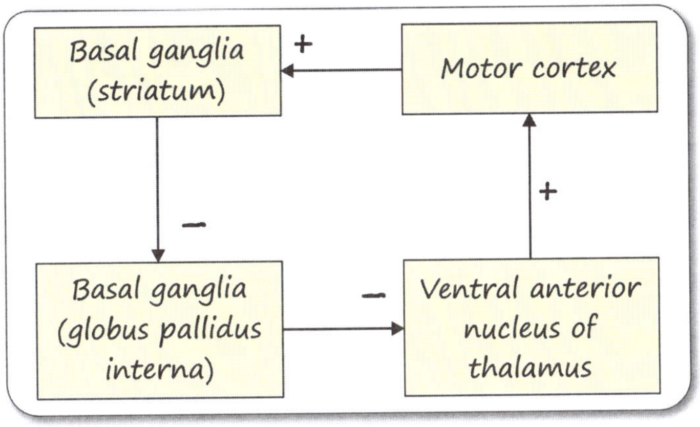

Direct Pathway-initiate voluntary movements

- To initiate voluntary movements, motor cortex must inhibit basal ganglia
- Motor cortex does this through activating striatum.
- Striatum inhibits Globus pallidus interna (GPi) by releasing the neurotransmitter GABA
- Since the GPi is inhibited, it cannot inhibit Ventral Anterior (VA) nucleus of thalamus (Disinhibition)
- VA nucleus of thalamus can now activate motor cortex for all voluntary movements to occur

Indirect Pathway

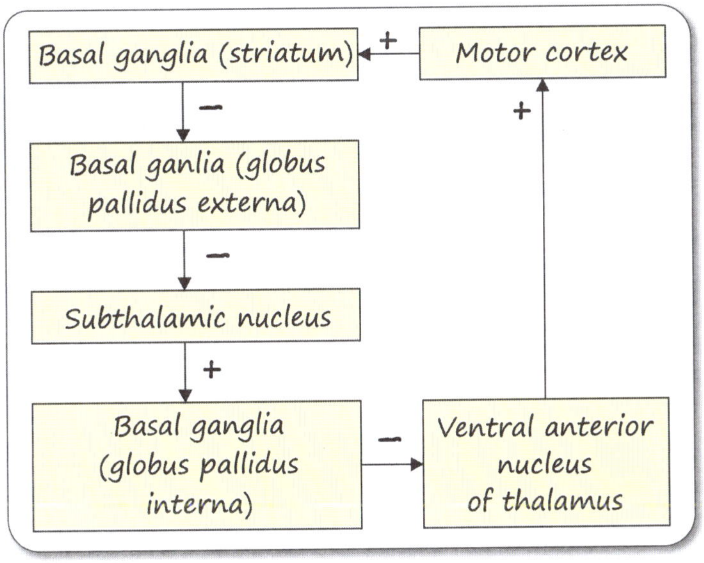

Indirect Pathway—terminate the initiated movement

- To terminate the motor movement once it is initiated Globus pallidus interna (GPi) must be activated again. Remember GPi is inhibited in direct pathway
- GPi is activated by subthalamic nucleus
- But, subt halamic nucleus is tonically inhibited by Globus pallidus Externa (GPe)
- Now to inhibit GPe, motor cortex activates st riatum
- Striatum inhibits GPe. Now, the subthalamic nucleus is activated
- Subthalamic nucleus activates Globus pallidus interna (GPi) which further inhibits Ventral Anterior (VA) nucleus of thalamus—terminate the initiated movement

MUST KNOW

Role of Dopamine: Dopamine activates direct pathway and inhibits indirect pathway. Dopamine activates direct pathway through D_1 receptor. Dopamine inhibits indirect pathway through D_2 receptor. Ultimately, by doing this, **dopamine facilitates voluntary motor movements.**

Involuntary movements and related lesions

Involuntary movement	Lesion
Rest tremor—due to regular, alternating 8-Hz contractions of antagonistic muscles	Substantia nigra pars compacta (SNc)
Chorea	Caudate nucleus
Athetosis	Globus pallidus
Hemiballismus	Subthalamic Nucleus

THALAMUS

Thalamic nuclei and their functions

Thalamic nuclei	Functions
Lateral geniculate bodies	• Concerned with vision
Medial geniculate bodies	• Concerned with hearing
Ventral posterior lateral (VPL) and ventral posteromedial nuclei (VPM)	• Transmit somatosensory information to sensory cortex
Ventral anterior and ventral lateral nuclei	• Concerned with motor functions • Receive input from basal ganglia and cerebellum • Project to the motor cortex
Anterior nuclei	• Forms part of Papez circuit concerned with learning and memory
Midline and intralaminar nuclei	• Nonspecific thalamic nuclei having widespread projections
Dorsomedial thalamic nucleus	• Concerned with olfaction (smell)

HYPOTHALAMUS

Hypothalamic nuclei along with their functions

Hypothalamic nuclei	Functions
Anterior	Responds to heat
Posterior	Responds to cold
Lateral	Feeding center
Ventromedial	Satiety center
Suprachiasmatic	Circadian rhythm
Supraoptic	Vasopressin (ADH)
Paraventricular	Oxytocin
Preoptic	Sleep center
Mammillary bodies	Learning and memory

LEARNING AND MEMORY

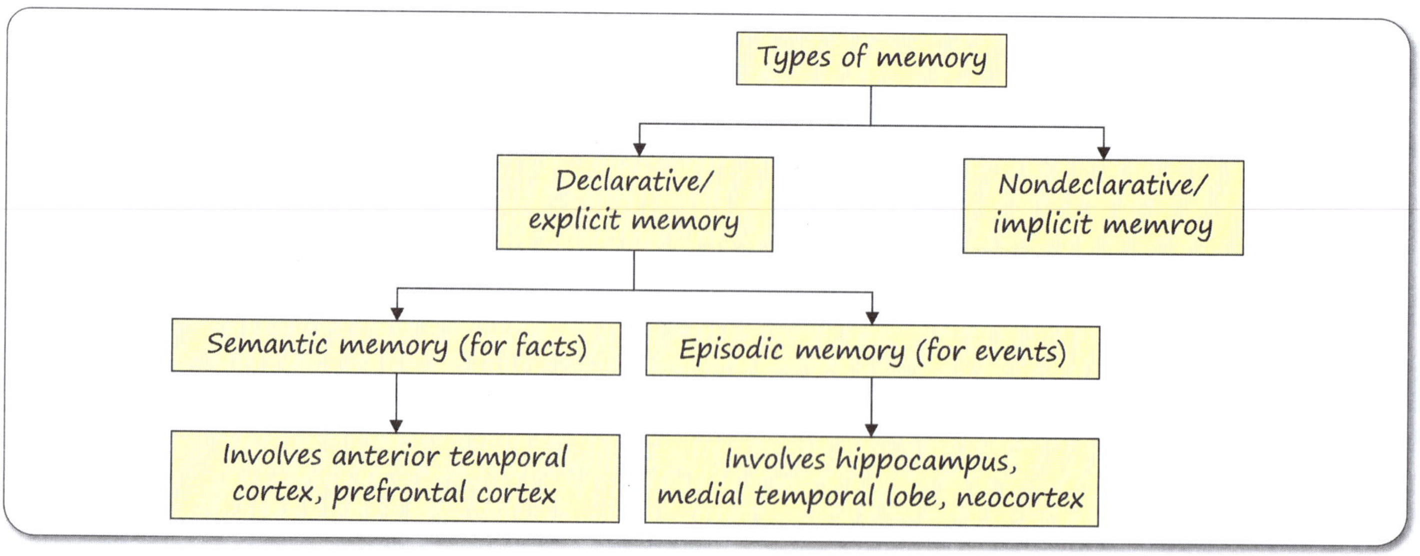

Types of memory

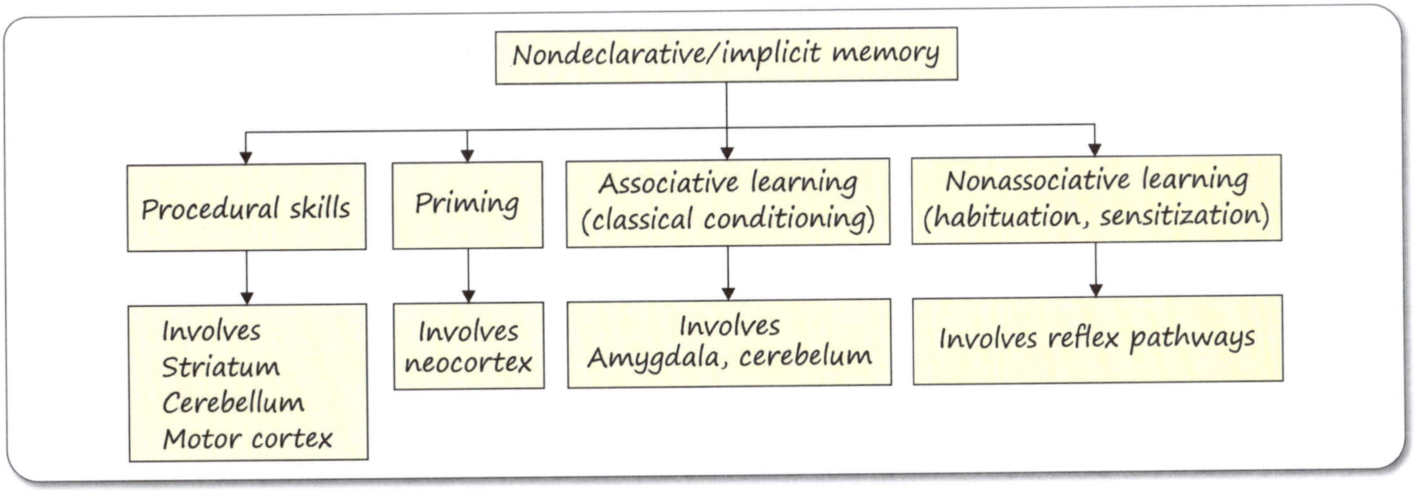

Types of nondeclarative/implicit memory

Types of memory based on time:

- **Short-term memory:** Lasts for seconds to hours.
- **Working memory**: A form of short-term memory which stores information temporarily.
- **Long-term memory:** Stores memories for years. Such stored memories are also called "**Engram**".

Role of Hippocampus in Learning and Memory

- Conversion of short-term memory into long-term memory. This function is also called consolidation or Long-Term Potentiation (LTP).
- According to Hebb's rule, if one neuron excites another neuron repeatedly and persistently, the synapse between those two neurons strengthens. This is seen as conversion of short-term memory into long-term memory in hippocampal neurons.
- Neurotransmitter concerned with LTP in hippocampus is Glutamate.
- **Nitric oxide** released from the postsynaptic neuron also increases glutamate release that helps in LTP.
- **Hippocampal lesions** will have problem in converting short-term memory into long-term memory—**Anterograde amnesia**

In long-term depression, synapse between two neurons weakens. It has a role in learning and memory. Long-term depression happens mainly in cerebellum.

Other Brain Areas Concerned with Learning and Memory

- **Mammillary bodies:** Forms a part of Papez circuit concerned with learning and memory. Lesions in this area cause Wernicke-Korsakoff syndrome.
- **Anterior nucleus of thalamus:** Here, lesion causes loss of recent memory.
- **Basal Forebrain—Nucleus basalis of Meynert**—Fibers containing **acetylcholine** project to hippocampus. Loss of these fibers occurs in **Alzheimer's disease.**
- **Amygdala:** It is concerned with emotionally-related memories.
- **Corpus callosum:** Hemispheric transfer of memory occurs through this part.

LANGUAGE AND SPEECH

- **Broca's area:** Located in left inferior frontal gyrus (Brodmann areas 44). It is the motor area for speech responsible for vocalization. Lesion-Broca's Aphasia—Reduced speech output. Impaired repetition (Non-Fluent Aphasia).
- **Wernicke's area:** Located at posterior end of the superior temporal gyrus (Brodmann area 22). It is the sensory area for speech responsible for comprehension. Lesion—**Wernicke's** Aphasia-Impaired comprehension. Speaks a lot without any meaning (Fluent Aphasia).
- **Arcuate fasciculus:** It is the bidirectional pathway through which Wernicke's area communicates with Broca's area. Lesion-Conduction Aphasia.
- **Angular gyrus (Brodmann area 39):** Process information from words that are read (visual information). Lesion-Anomic Aphasia (cannot name what they see).

CEREBRAL BLOOD FLOW

- Around 750 mL/min or 15% of cardiac output.
- O_2 consumption—20% of the total body resting O_2 consumption.

- Regulation:
  - **Autoregulation:** Blood flow constant despite change in pressure (65–140 mm Hg)
  - **Hypercarbia:** Increases cerebral blood flow
  - **Hypothermia:** Reduction of body temperature by 1°C decreases cerebral blood flow by 7%. Therapeutic hypothermia is useful in neurosurgical procedures to minimize blood loss.

CEREBROSPINAL FLUID

- **Volume of cerebrospinal fluid (CSF) is 150 mL**
- **Rate of CSF production is 550 mL/day**
- **CSF turnover is 3.7 times a day.**
- **Normal CSF pressure is 70–180 mm H_2O**

Compared with plasma, CSF has **high** concentrations of:

- Chloride
- Magnesium
- Sodium

Concentration **equal** in CSF and plasma:

- Osmolality
- Bicarbonate ions

Compared with plasma, CSF has **low** concentrations of:

- Glucose (2/3rd of plasma glucose)
- Proteins

β_2-Transferrin, a product of neuraminidase activity, is very specific for CSF. It is found only in CSF. It is a CSF marker. In CSF rhinorrhea and CSF otorrhea, the leaking fluid tests positive for β_2-Transferrin.

ELECTROENCEPHALOGRAPHY WAVES

Electroencephalography (EEG) waves along with their frequencies and characteristics

EEG wave	Frequency	Characteristics
Alpha wave	8–13 Hz	• Are most prominent over parieto occipital areas • Seen when the patient is resting with the eyes closed • **Alpha block** – When attention is diverted, the alpha rhythm is replaced by fast, irregular low-voltage activity
Beta wave	14–30 Hz	• Are most prominent over parieto frontal areas • Seen during wakefulness
Theta wave	4–7 Hz	• Generated in hippocampus • Pathologically seen often in degenerative brain diseases
Delta wave	<4 Hz	• Seen in very deep sleep
Gamma wave	30–80 Hz	• Seen during focused attention

Contd...

SLEEP

Sleep is subdivided into two phases, which are **non-rapid eye movement (NREM) sleep and rapid eye movement (REM) sleep.**

Non-rapid Eye Movement Sleep (NREM)

- **Comprises 4 stages:** Stage 1, Stage 2, Stage 3 Stage 4
- **Stage 1 NREM (N1):** Transition between waking and sleep. EEG shows low frequency (4–7 Hz) theta waves.
- **Stage 2 NREM (N2):** Waves with frequency 12–14 Hz, called sleep spindles, are seen. High voltage biphasic waves, called K complexes, are also seen.
- **Stage 3 and 4 NREM (N3):** Deepest sleep. Delta waves appear >50% of the time in the EEG.
- NREM sleep occupies approximately 75% of the total sleep time. Stage 2 NREM occupies the maximum duration (45%) followed by Stages 3 and 4 (25%) and least is Stage 1 (5%).

NREM sleep is characterized by decrease in body movements, heart rate, breathing—Respiration becomes slow and regular, blood pressure, metabolic rate, temperature decrease.

- REM sleep is accompanied by increase in blood pressure, heart rate and metabolism.
- Spontaneous penile erection is experienced by men. Women experience sexual arousal.

Rapid Eye Movement (REM) Sleep

- Also called superficial sleep, active sleep and paradoxical sleep.
- Called paradoxical sleep because EEG resembles like that of an awake individual (beta waves).
- PGO spikes—Called **pontogeniculo-occipital (PGO) spikes.** These large phasic potentials are highly characteristic of REM sleep.
- **Electrooculography (EOG) shows eyeball movements during REM sleep.**
- During REM sleep—Muscle atonia. Electromyography (EMG)—No activity
- Muscles that do not undergo atonia during REM sleep are extraocular muscles and diaphragm.

Endocrine Hormone Changes during Sleep

- Growth hormone level rises in stages 3 and 4 NREM sleep.
- Prolactin level rises during REM sleep.
- Around the time of puberty, there is increase in nocturnal LH secretion.
- Sleep onset is associated with inhibition of thyroid-stimulating hormone (TSH) and ACTH.
- Pineal hormone melatonin—Secreted predominantly at night. Melatonin is the N-acetylated product of serotonin found in the pineal gland. MT_1 receptor of melatonin—Promotes sleep. **Melatonin Agonist Ramelteon is** useful in the treatment of insomnia.

Neural areas and neurotransmitters that promote wakefulness

Wakefulness promoting brain areas	Neurotransmitter involved	Neurotransmitter levels during NREM sleep	Neurotransmitter levels during REM sleep
Cholinergic nuclei of pons-midbrain junction	Acetylcholine	Decrease	**Increase** (REM-ON) **Responsible for PGO spikes**
Locus coeruleus	Norepinephrine	Decrease	Decrease
Raphe nuclei	Serotonin	Decrease	Decrease
Tuberomammillary nuclei	Histamine	Decrease	Decrease
Lateral hypothalamus	Orexin	Decrease	Decrease

Parasomnias

Non-rapid eye movement sleep parasomnias	Rapid eye movement sleep parasomnias
• Sleepwalking (Somnambulism)—Commonly arises from NREM stages 3 and 4 • Sleep Talking • Sleep Bruxism—NREM stage 2 • Sleep enuresis (Bed wetting) • Sleep Terrors (Pavor Nocturnus)	• Narcolepsy—Occurs due to the loss of orexinergic neurons from lateral hypothalamus. Treatment is CNS stimulants like Modafinil and Sodium oxybate—improves alertness • Nightmares

5. RESPIRATORY PHYSIOLOGY

LUNG AIRWAY GENERATIONS–WEIBEL'S MODEL OF AIRWAYS

- Lung airways are divided into 23 generations out of which:
  1. First 16 generations—Conducting airways
  2. Last 7 generations—Exchange (respiratory) airways

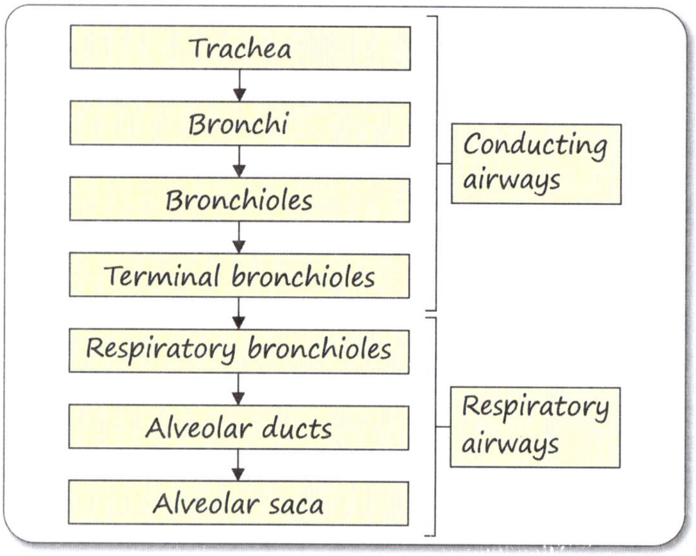

Conducting Airways

- Have no role in exchange of gases. The air present in conductions airways is called dead space ventilation. It is around 150 mL.
- Airways with highest airway resistance are the medium-sized bronchi.
- Lining epithelium—Pseudostratified ciliated columnar epithelium.
- Cilia beat toward the nasopharynx ("mucociliary escalator")—Helps in clearing sputum.
- Cilia move because of the dynein: If dynein arm is absent, then cilia become immotile. Seen in Kartagener syndrome characterized by the triad of recurrent sinusitis, bronchiectasis and situs inversus (Cilia is responsible for rotation of internal organs during development).
- Ciliary immotility because of thick secretions seen in Cystic fibrosis (CF)—mutation in Cystic fibrosis transmembrane conductance regulator (CFTR)-chloride channel
- Cells present in conducting airways:
  - Basal cells: Function as the stem cell
  - Clara cells: Also called club cells. Function as the stem cell
  - Neuroepithelial cells-neuroepithelial bodies (NEBs). Sensors of oxygen. Contains serotonin. They are also called Kulchitsky cells. Carcinoid tumor of lung called Kulchitsky cell carcinoma arises from them.

MUST KNOW

Airway Smooth Muscles

- Mainly seen in conducting airways
- Can undergo constriction (Bronchoconstriction) or dilation (Bronchodilation)
- Bronchial smooth muscles are under the control of both neural (autonomic nervous system) and chemicals.
- Airway smooth muscle contraction contributes to the airway narrowing (bronchospasm) in disease conditions like asthma.

Agents that modify bronchial smooth muscle activity	
Bronchoconstriction	**Bronchodilation**
• Parasympathetic stimulation • Acetylcholine • Histamine • Leukotrienes **(most potent (bronchoconstrictor)**	• Sympathetic stimulation (β_2 receptors) • Circulating β_2 agonists • Nitric oxide

Respiratory (Alveolar) Airways

- Comprises the last 7 generations of airways where gas exchange occurs.

Two types of alveolar epithelial cells are seen as follows:

1. **Alveolar epithelial cells—type I:** Flat cells that cover around 95% of alveolar epithelial surface area.
2. **Alveolar epithelial cells—type II:** These are the stem cells from which type I cells arise. Occupy only 5% of alveolar epithelial surface area but they represent 60% of the epithelial cells in the alveoli. Also called granular pneumocytes. Most important function of type II cell is the production of **surfactant.**

PULMONARY SURFACTANT

Composition of surfactant	
Surfactant lipids	**Surfactant proteins**
• Account for approximately 90% of surfactant • Major surfactant lipids are: ▪ Dipalmitoyl phosphatidylcholine (DPPC)–Lecithin—most abundant component of surfactant ▪ Phosphatidylglycerol	• Account for approximately 90% of surfactant • Major surfactant proteins are: ▪ Surfactant protein-A (SP-A) ▪ Surfactant protein-B (SP-B) ▪ Surfactant protein-C (SP-C) ▪ Surfactant protein-D (SP-D)

- After synthesis, surfactant is stored inside alveolar type II cells in the form of **lamellar bodies** prior to release.
- Surfactant reduces the surface tension. This action prevents alveolar collapse during expiration (atelectasis) and makes alveoli more compliant.
- Surfactant proteins (SP- A & SP –D) play a role in lung immunity.
- Surfactant levels are useful to assess fetal lung maturity.
- Lecithin/sphingomyelin (L/S) ratio ≥2 indicates lung maturity.
- **Shake test:** Also called Bubble test or Clement's test. This test is based on the ability of pulmonary surfactant to form a foam or bubble on shaking.
- Surfactant production is accelerated by glucocorticoids and thyroid hormones.
- Surfactant production is inhibited by high levels of insulin, long-term inhalation of 100% O_2, smoking.

MUST KNOW

Deficiency of pulmonary surfactant leads to Hyaline membrane disease. Also called Respiratory Distress Syndrome (RDS). Treatment is **Surfactant replacement therapy by exogenous surfactant drugs like beractant.**

MECHANICS OF BREATHING

- This is about the processes that involve taking in air (inspiration) and giving out (expiration).
- This air movement is governed by Boyle's Law which states that "at constant temperature, pressure (P) of a gas is inversely related to its volume (V)".

Important pressures in respiration are intrapleural pressure, alveolar pressure and transpulmonary pressure.

1. Intrapleural pressure

- Normal intrapleural pressure is negative (sub atmospheric) around –2.5 mm Hg at the start of inspiration.
- Chest wall always tries to expand. The natural tendency of lung is always to collapse. When these two opposite forces pull on the intrapleural space, a negative pressure (Vacuum) is created. This is the **cause for Negativity of Intrapleural Pressure.**

Intrapleural pressure changes	
At the beginning of normal inspiration	–2.5 mm Hg
During normal inspiration	–6 mm Hg
At the end of forceful inspiration	–30 mm Hg
At the end of forced expiration	+50 mm Hg

2. Alveolar pressure

- Alveolar pressure is exactly equal to the atmospheric pressure at rest.
- It becomes negative during inspiration. Logically, this decrease in alveolar pressure is what brings air from environment into the lung.

Alveolar pressure changes	
At rest	Equal to atmospheric pressure (0 mm Hg)
During normal inspiration	–1 mm Hg
At the end of normal inspiration	Zero (0)
During normal expiration	+1 mm Hg
At the end of normal expiration	Zero (0)

3. Transpulmonary pressure

- Transpulmonary pressure = Alveolar pressure – intrapleural pressure

MUSCLES OF INSPIRATION AND EXPIRATION

Pressure changes are aided by contraction of certain muscles to aid the movement of air inside and out of the lung.

- **Muscles of inspiration:** Diaphragm–major muscle for inspiration, external intercostal muscle, Scalene, Sternocleidomastoid.
- **Muscles of expiration:** Expiration is largely a passive process at rest. Because of the elastic nature of lung, it recoils itself during expiration. Active expiration occurs during exercise. Muscles of active expiration are rectus abdominis, external and internal oblique muscles, transversus abdominis, internal intercostal muscles.

PRESSURE VOLUME RELATIONSHIP IN LUNG—THE CONCEPT OF "COMPLIANCE"

- During inspiration, alveoli distend. This distension force is Compliance.
- This distension will be opposed by two opposing forces namely elastic recoil forces and surface tension forces. This surface tension force is held in check by surfactant.
- Compliance is defined as "the change in volume per unit change in the pressure".
- Compliance = $\Delta V/\Delta P$
- Compliance of lung is 0.2 L/cm water

There are three types of compliance namely Static compliance, Dynamic compliance and Specific compliance.

1. Static compliance is the compliance measured when breathing does not take place.
2. Dynamic compliance is the compliance measured when the subject is breathing. Airway resistance (Impedance to airflow) is considered here.
3. Specific compliance = Compliance/Functional residual capacity (FRC).

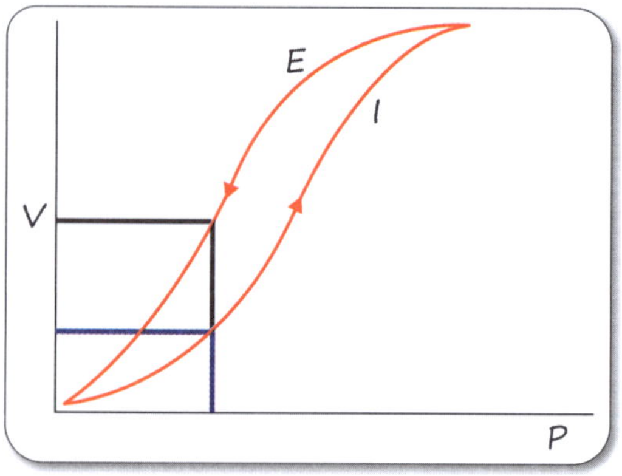

Lung compliance

MUST KNOW

Important points to be noted in compliance curve are:

- The curve has inspiratory (I) and expiratory (E) components
- Note that the inspiratory and expiratory compliance curves do not coincide. This difference is called hysteresis
- Compliance is the slope $\Delta V/\Delta P$
- The lung volume at any given pressure is greater during expiration than during inspiration
- Compliance is greatest at mid pressure range
- At high pressures, compliance is lowest (curve flattens)

PRESSURE VOLUME CURVES OF LUNG (P_L), CHEST WALL (P_W), LUNG AND CHEST WALL COMBINED (P_{TR})

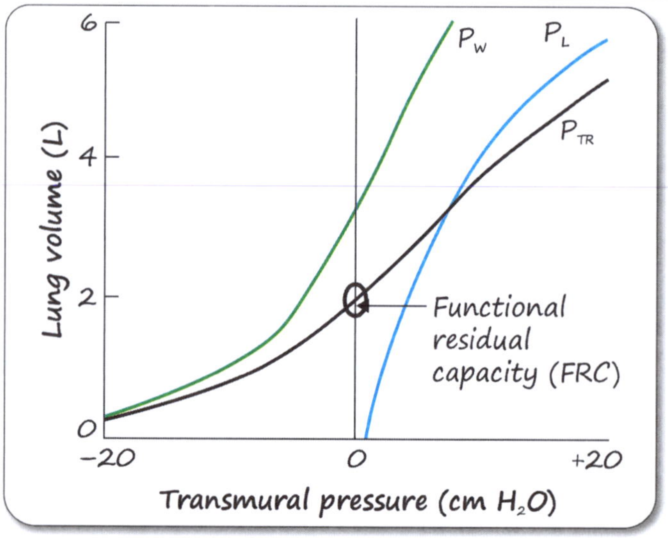

Pressure-Volume Curves

- At rest, lung volume is at functional residual capacity (FRC)—the circled point in graph
- The system is relaxed at rest meaning that the inward recoil of lung is balanced by the outward expansion of chest wall (equilibrium point)
- FRC is also called "relaxation volume" or "equilibrium volume"
- If lung was allowed to recoil without the chest wall in expiration at zero pressure the lung is at its MINIMAL VOLUME, which is below residual volume

MUST KNOW

- Condition causing increase in compliance: Emphysema
- Conditions causing decrease in compliance: Pulmonary fibrosis, interstitial lung diseases

LUNG VOLUMES AND CAPACITIES

- Lung volumes and capacities can be either static or dynamic
- These are usually recorded on a spirometer. The recording is called **Spirogram.**

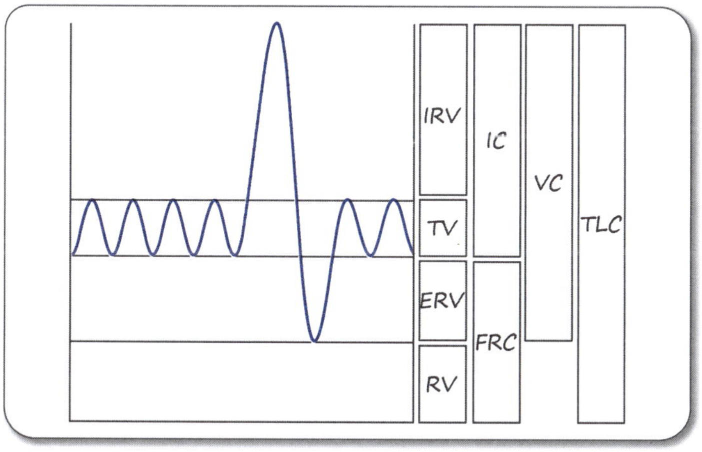

Static lung volume and capacities

Static lung volumes and their normal values

Static lung volumes	Normal value
Tidal volume (TV)	500–750 mL
Inspiratory reserve volume (IRV)	3000 mL (2000–3200 mL)
Expiratory reserve volume (ERV)	1200 mL
Residual volume (RV) It is the volume of air left in lungs after forceful expiration. Residual volume (RV) is usually around 20% of total lung capacity (TLC)	1300 mL

Static lung capacities and their normal values

Static lung capacities	Normal value
Inspiratory capacity (IC) = TV + IRV	3500 mL
Functional residual capacity (FRC) = RV + ERV It is the amount of air remaining in the lungs after a **normal tidal expiration**	2500 mL
Vital capacity (VC) = IRV + TV + ERV	4700 mL
Total lung capacity (TLC) = IRV + TV + ERV + RV	5900 mL

Contd...

- Lung volumes and capacities that cannot be measured by spirometry are:
  - Residual volume (RV)
  - Functional residual capacity (FRC)
  - Total lung capacity (TLC)
- They are usually measured by:
  - Helium dilution technique
  - Nitrogen washout technique
  - Body plethysmography

Dynamic Lung Volume and Capacities

- For these measurements, time factor is considered.
- They are measured using spirometry with the help of **flow volume loop.**

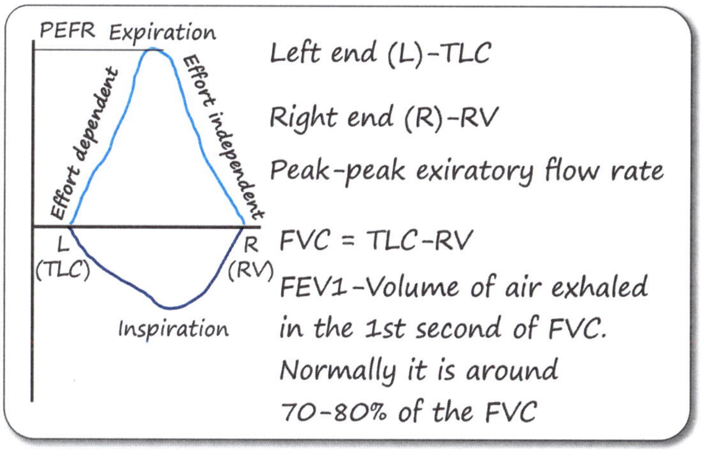

Flow volume loop

- **Effort dependent part of the curve**
  - It is the part of the curve from total lung capacity (TLC) to peak expiratory flow (PEF).
  - This part of the curve depends on the expiratory effort, the velocity and the force of the expiratory muscle contraction.
- **Effort independent part of the curve**
  - It is the part of the curve from peak expiratory flow (PEF) to residual volume (RV).
  - This part of the curve is relatively effort-independent and it reflects the peripheral airway resistance and lung elastic recoil. Usually affected in chronic obstructive pulmonary disease (COPD).

FEV_1/FVC Ratio

- FEV1/FVC ratio is also called **Tiffeneau index.**
- Normally, the FEV_1/FVC ratio is greater than 70%
- This ratio is used to differentiate obstructive from restrictive lung disorders.

FEV_1/FVC Ratio	
Obstructive lung diseases	Restrictive lung diseases
• FEV_1/FVC Ratio is **low** because FEV_1 drops much more significantly than FVC	• FEV_1/FVC Ratio remains **normal** if the drop in FVC is proportional to drop in FEV_1 • FEV_1/FVC Ratio may **increase** if the FVC drops more markedly than FEV_1

VENTILATION AND PERFUSION

Ventilation (V)

- Out of the 500 mL of tidal volume we take in, only 350 mL of air reaches alveoli (Alveolar ventilation) and the remaining 150 mL is dead space ventilation.

Environmental air composition	
Gas	Percentage
Nitrogen	79%
Oxygen	20.95%
Carbon dioxide	0.04%
Atmospheric pressure at sea level is 760 mm Hg	

MUST KNOW

- Partial pressure of oxygen in environmental air is 760 *21/100 = 160 mm Hg
- Partial pressure of oxygen in inspired air is 150 mm Hg
- Partial pressure of oxygen in alveolar air is 100 mm Hg
- Partial pressure of oxygen in expired air is 120 mm Hg. This contains 16% oxygen. Mouth to mouth breathing provides 16% oxygen.

- The partial pressure of oxygen in alveolar air can be found out using **"Alveolar Gas Equation" which is as follows:**

$$PAO_2 = PIO_2 - \frac{PACO_2}{R}$$

- In the equation, PAO_2 is the partial pressure of oxygen in alveolar air, PIO_2 is the partial pressure of oxygen in the inspired air, $PACO_2$ is the partial pressure of carbon dioxide in alveolar air, R is the respiratory exchange ratio—which is the ratio of CO_2 produced by oxygen consumed.

Alveolar Ventilation

- Out of the 500 mL of tidal volume, only 350 mL reaches alveoli.
- For a respiratory rate of 12 breaths/min, alveolar ventilation is 12 *(500−350) = 4.2 L/min
- Alveolar ventilation and $PACO_2$ are inversely related if CO_2 production is constant. If alveolar ventilation is doubled, then alveolar PCO_2 ($PACO_2$) will be reduced to half.

Dead Space Ventilation

- Dead space ventilation means the ventilation that is not used for gas exchange.
- It can be of three types, anatomic dead space, alveolar dead space, physiologic or total dead space.
  - Anatomic dead space is the volume of air present in the conducting zone (first 16 generations) which is not used for gas exchange—150 mL
  - Alveolar dead space is the volume of air present in those alveoli which do not take part in gas exchange. In healthy individuals, its value is zero.
  - Physiologic dead space = anatomic dead space + alveolar dead space
- In healthy individuals, physiologic dead space roughly equals anatomic dead space.
- ***Measurement of anatomic dead space:*** single-breath Nitrogen method, also called ***Fowler's*** method.
- Physiologic dead space is measured with the help of an equation termed **Bohr's equation.**

Bohr's equation

$$V_D = V_T \times \frac{PACO_2 - PECO_2}{PACO_2}$$

- Here, in this equation, V_D is the dead space ventilation, V_T is the tidal volume, $PECO_2$ is the partial pressure of CO_2 in mixed expired air and $PACO_2$ is the alveolar $PACO_2$
- **V_D/V_T ratio:** This ratio is used to find out the proportion of ventilation remains in dead spaces. Normally the ratio is 150/500 which equals 0.3

Perfusion (Q)

- Perfusion is the pulmonary circulation around 5 L/min.
- The pulmonary vessel walls are thin compared to system vessels. They are highly distensible with large compliance.
- Pulmonary circulation is—"low-pressure, low-resistance and high capacitance system". This is to accommodate the cardiac output that lung receives for oxygenation of blood.
- Most important regulatory factor for pulmonary circulation is **hypoxia** (reduced PO_2).
- Hypoxia causes pulmonary vasoconstriction. This effect is different in systemic circulation where hypoxia causes vasodilation.
- Hypoxia inhibits an outward potassium current in pulmonary vascular smooth muscles leading to depolarization. This is due to direct effect of hypoxia.
- This depolarization opens calcium channels and entry of calcium ions.
- Calcium ions constrict vascular smooth muscles leading to vasoconstriction.
- Hypoxia-induced vasoconstriction diverts the blood from poorly ventilated regions (hypoxic) to well-ventilated regions of the lung for effective oxygenation.
- Depending on the relationship between alveolar pressure (P_A), pulmonary arterial pressure (Pa) and pulmonary venous pressure (Pv), the lung blood flow can be divided into three zones.

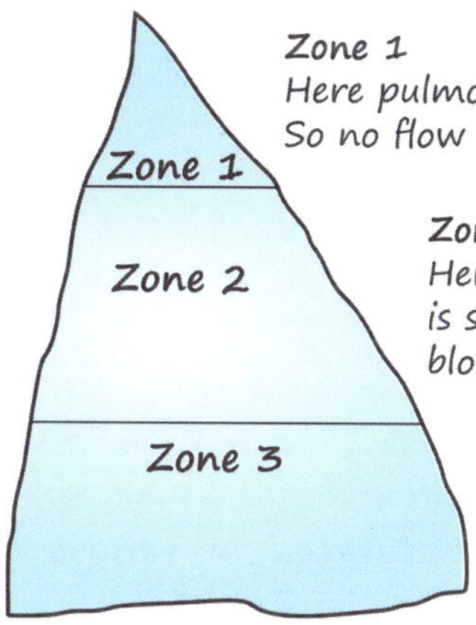

Zone 1
Here pulmonary arterial pressure falls below alveolar pressure and the capillaries are closed. So no flow is possible in zone 1 (no flow zone)-$P_A > P_a > P_v$ Zone 1 is seen in the apex of lung

Zone 2
Here pulmonary arterial pressure exceeds alveolar pressure but the venous pressure is still less than alveolar pressure-$P_a > P_A > P_v$ Zone 2 is characterized by intermittent blood flow (waterfall effect). Zone 2 is seen in the middle part of lung

Zone 3
Zone occurs when the pulmonary artery pressure exceeds the pulmonary venous pressure which exceeds the alveolar pressure ($P_a > P_v > P_A$). Zone 3 is characterized by continuous blood flow. Zone 3 is seen in the base of lung

Pulmonary circulation–Lung zones

Ventilation Perfusion (V/Q) Ratio

MUST KNOW

- V/Q ratio = Alveolar ventilation/Pulmonary circulation = 4.2/5.5 = 0.8
- V/Q ratio = 4.2/5.5 = 0.8
- V/Q ratio is more at the apex of lung (3.3)
- V/Q ratio is less at the base of lung (0.6)

- High PO_2 of the apical regions of lung favors the growth of mycobacterium tuberculosis.
- **Ventilation–Perfusion ratio (V/Q ratio) = Zero (O)**
  - This means that ventilation (numerator) is zero. So, the ratio becomes zero.
  - Physiological cause of non-uniform ventilation: Shunt blood perfused regions–Oxygenation of shunt blood does not occur because there is no ventilation.
  - Pathological causes of non-uniform ventilation: Collapse of lung (emphysema), foreign body obstruction.
- **Ventilation–Perfusion ratio (V/Q ratio) = ∞ (Infinity)**
  - This means that the perfusion is nil (denominator). So, the ratio becomes infinity.
  - Physiological cause of nonuniform perfusion: Dead spaces—No gas exchange
  - Pathological causes of nonuniform perfusion: Pulmonary embolism, compression of pulmonary vessels by high alveolar pressures, tumor occluding pulmonary vessels.

DIFFUSION OF GASES

- Gases move into and out of the alveoli using a transport process called **simple diffusion.**
- Diffusion means movement of molecules from an area of high concentration to area of low concentration. It is passive process. It does not require any energy for transport of substances.

MUST KNOW

The law that governs the diffusion of gases in lung is called **Fick's law. According to this law, diffusion of gases is directly proportional to concentration gradient, area of respiratory membrane and inversely proportional to thickness of membrane.**

- Diffusion of gases is also directly proportional to lipid solubility but inversely proportional to size of the molecules.
- In clinical practice, carbon monoxide is the gas of choice for measuring diffusion capacity because it is the diffusion limited gas. The procedure is called diffusing capacity of the lung for carbon monoxide or DLCO
- Normal value of DLCO is 25 mL/min/mm Hg
- Diffusion coefficient of O_2 is about 1.23 times that of CO. So, diffusing capacity for oxygen is 25 * 1.23 = 30 mL/min/mm Hg

MUST KNOW

- **Conditions that increase diffusion capacity (DLCO) are** exercise, polycythemia, alveolar hemorrhage.

Contd...

- **Conditions that decrease diffusion capacity (DLCO) are** emphysema, pulmonary fibrosis, anemia.

TRANSPORT OF GASES

- Once the oxygen diffuses from alveoli into the pulmonary capillaries, it is carried to the left heart and from there oxygen is transported in blood to all other body regions.
- Due to metabolism of oxygen by tissues, carbon dioxide is produced and it is transported in blood to the lungs for expelling it out of the body.

OXYGEN TRANSPORT

- Oxygen is transported in blood in two forms: Dissolved form and combined with hemoglobin (major form).
- **Each gram of hemoglobin transports 1.34 mL of oxygen.**
- The hemoglobin concentration in normal blood is about 15 g/dL. Therefore, 1 dL of blood contains (1.34 mL × 15) 20.1 mL of oxygen bound to hemoglobin.
- Arterial blood contains around 19.8 mL of O_2 per dL, out of which 0.29 mL is in dissolved form and 19.5 mL is bound to hemoglobin.
- **Hemoglobin is 75% saturated in venous blood and its oxygen content is 15.2 mL/dL.**
- Binding and release of oxygen from hemoglobin is assessed using **oxygen-hemoglobin dissociation curve (ODC).**

Oxygen Dissociation Curve

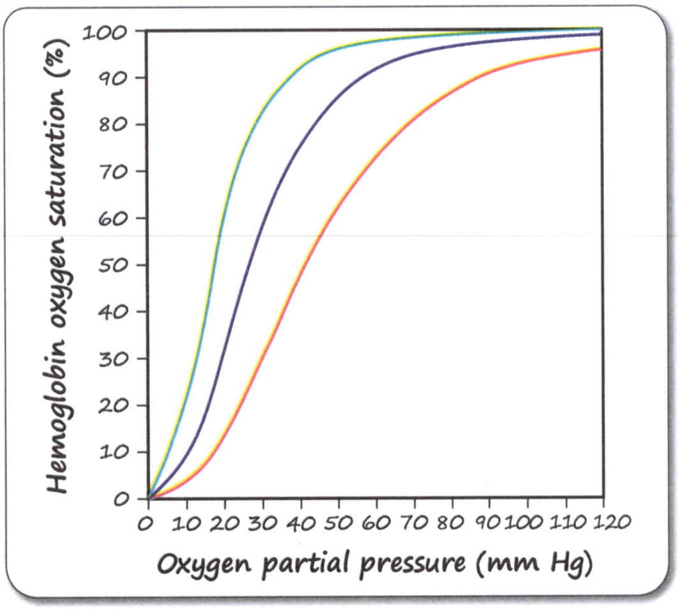

- X-axis—Partial pressure of oxygen (PO_2), Y-axis - Percentage O_2 saturation of Hb. The curve is sigmoid shaped
- P_{50}—is the partial pressure of oxygen at which hemoglobin saturation with oxygen is 50%. The value of P_{50} is around 25-27 mm Hg
- Hemoglobin affinity for O_2 is inversely related to the P_{50} value
- Once the first molecule of oxygen binds with the first heme in Hb, it increases the affinity for further oxygen binding
- **Affinity for the fourth O_2 molecule is the highest**
- This is termed cooperative binding kinetics and it is the reason for the sigmoid nature of the curve
- Curve can be shifted either to right side or left side

- *ODC shift to right means there is decreased affinity of oxygen to hemoglobin leading to release of oxygen (unloading of oxygen). It happens in tissues.*

Oxygen Dissociation Curve–Right Shift

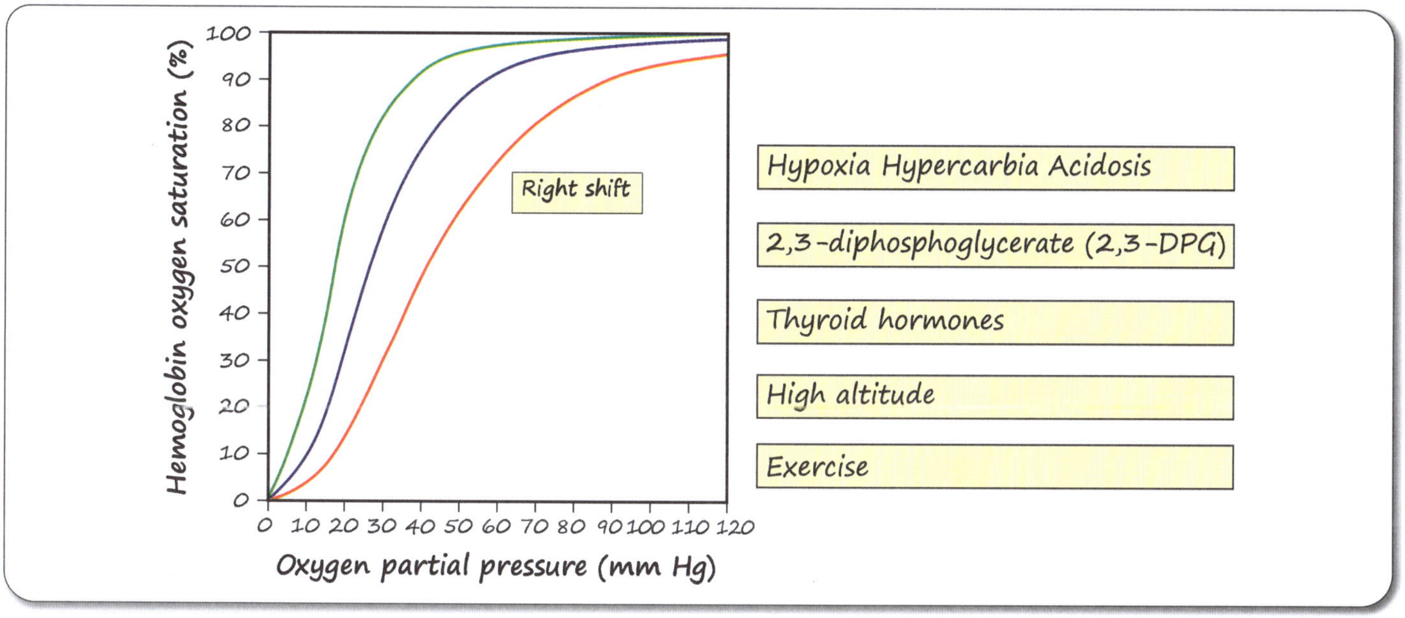

- *ODC shift to left means there is increased affinity of oxygen to hemoglobin leading to loading of oxygen. It happens in lungs.*

Oxygen Dissociation Curve–Left Shift

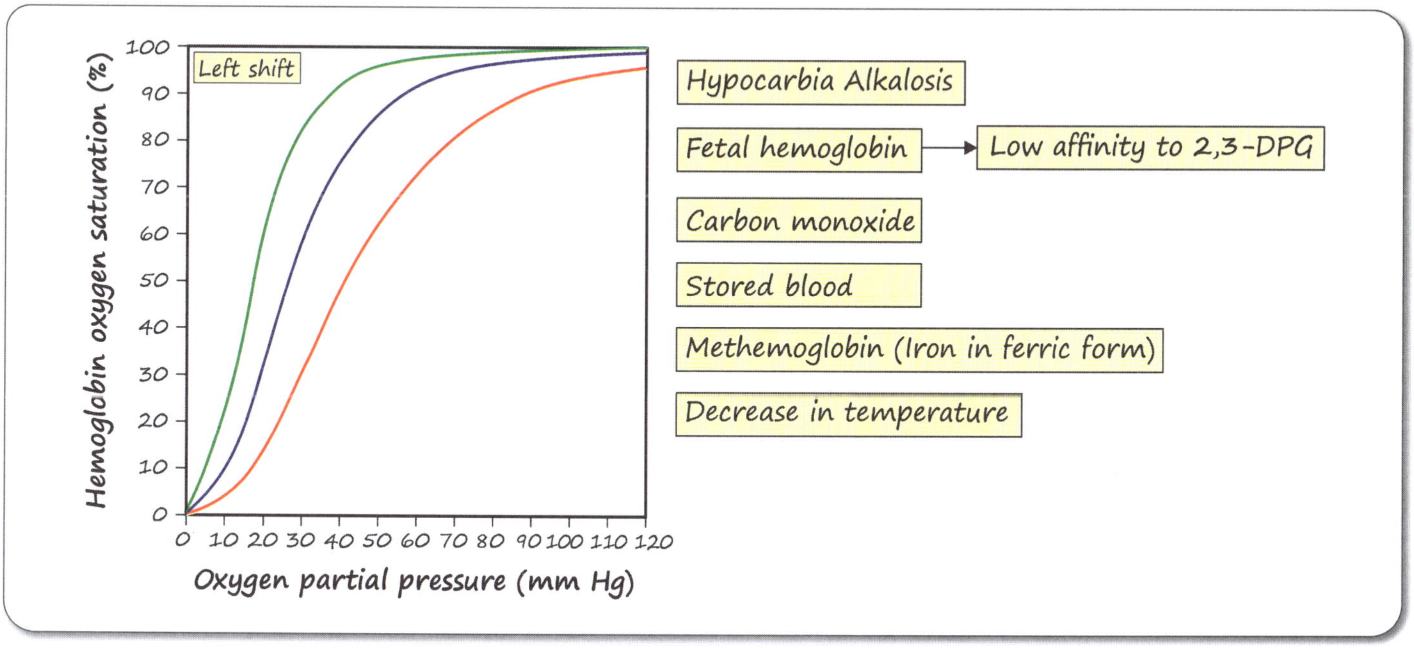

- The decrease in O_2 affinity of hemoglobin when pH of blood falls (PCO_2 rises) is called the **Bohr effect.** This leads to release of oxygen at tissues.
- Double Bohr effect occurs at the fetal-maternal interface in placenta.
- Haldane effect states that "when oxygen binds with hemoglobin, carbon dioxide is released at lungs and when oxygen is released from hemoglobin, carbon dioxide is loaded at tissues".

TRANSPORT OF CARBON DIOXIDE

- CO_2 is transported as bicarbonate form (70%—the major form of CO_2 transport) and as carbamino compound form bound with hemoglobin.
- CO_2 is 20 times more soluble than O_2
- Total CO_2 content of arterial blood is 48 mL CO_2/100 mL
- Total CO_2 content of venous blood is 52 mL CO_2/100 mL
- In the normal operating range of **Carbon dioxide dissociation curve**, CO_2 content changes by around 4 mL/dL (52–48).
- **Chloride Shift**
  - Also called Hamburger phenomenon.
  - The channel responsible for chloride shift is called anion exchanger 1 (AE 1). It is also called Band 3 protein present in RBC membrane.
  - HCO_3—leaves the RBCs in exchange for Cl– (chloride shift) and is transported to the lungs in the plasma.
  - Cl^- ion is an osmotically active particle that drags water along with it into the RBCs.
  - Since RBCs take up water, it increases in size. This is the reason why hematocrit of venous blood is normally 3% greater than that of arterial blood.

REGULATION OF RESPIRATION

Respiratory regulation falls under two types, neural regulation of respiration and chemical regulation of respiration.

Neural Regulation of Respiration

- Respiration is both voluntary (cortical control) and involuntary (brain stem control).
- Brain stem areas that regulate breathing movements are:
  - **Medulla:** Generates the rhythm of respiration.
  - **Pons:** Fine tunes respiration by regulating the timings of inspiration and expiration.

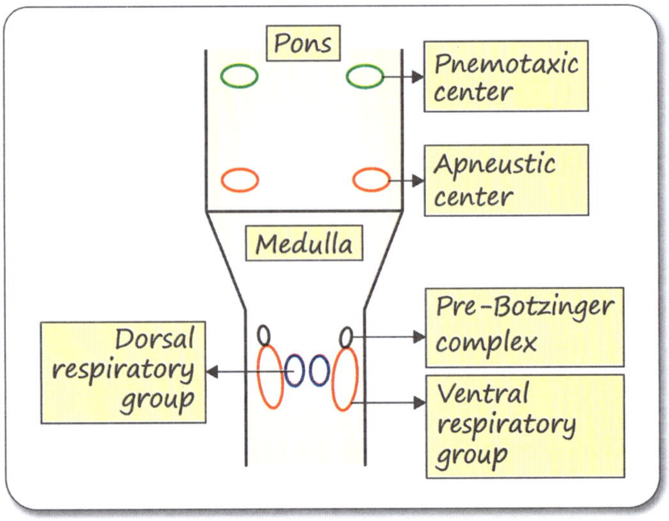

Neural areas regulating respiration

Brain area	Function
Pre-Botzinger complex	Pacemaker: initiates respiration
Pneumotaxic center	• Limits inspiration by inhibiting apneustic center. • Controls respiratory rate
Apneustic center	Prolong inspiration
Dorsal respiratory group	Generates RAMP signal for smooth increase in tidal volume during inspiration
Ventral respiratory group	Controls forceful expiration during exercise

- If vagus is cut, then respiration becomes slow and deep.
- Lesion below medulla—respiration stops.
- Pontomedullary junction lesion—pons and medulla are separated: Irregular respiration
- Mid pons lesion with vagus cut—pneumotaxic center separated from apneustic center: Inspiration is markedly prolonged. This breathing pattern is called **apneusis or inspiratory spasm.**

Respiratory Reflexes

Hering-Breuer Inflation Reflex

- Hering-Breuer Inflation reflex is atypical negative feedback reflex where "overinflation of lung inhibits further lung inflation".
- Receptors for this reflex are "slowly adapting receptors." Afferent information is carried by large myelinated fibers in the vagus.

- Protective reflex prevents overdistension of lung alveoli at larger tidal volumes (1500 mL).

Hering-Breuer Deflation Reflex

- Hering-Breuer deflation reflex is also a preventive reflex where "deflation of the lungs increases the ventilatory rate".
- Afferent information is carried by large myelinated fibers in the vagus.
- It is a protective reflex which helps prevent atelectasis (collapse) in conditions like pneumothorax.

The Paradoxical Reflex of Head

- The paradoxical reflex of head is paradoxical to **Hering-Breuer inflation reflex** where inflation of lungs causes further inflation.
- This reflex is the cause for lung inflation in newborn immediately after birth when the newborn takes the first breath.

J Receptor Reflex

- J receptors were discovered by an Indian physiologist A S Paintal.
- These receptors are located very close to the pulmonary capillaries (juxtapulmonary receptors).
- These receptors are the endings of slowly conducting unmyelinated vagal C fibers.
- J receptors are activated by increase in the interstitial fluid volume—pulmonary edema
- J receptor reflex is also called "Pulmonary chemoreflex".
- J receptor reflex response consists of rapid breathing, bradycardia and hypotension.

Altered Breathing Patterns (Periodic Breathing)

- **Cheyne-stokes respiration**
  - Characterized by periods of hyperpnea, hypopnea and apnea—waxing and waning
  - Normally occurs during sleep at high altitude
  - Also seen in congestive cardiac failure
- **Biot's breathing**
  - Characterized by periods of hyperpnea and apnea
  - Also called ataxic breathing: seen in damage to medulla and meningitis
- **Kussmaul respiration**
  - Hyperventilation characterized by regular, deep, fast respiration
  - Commonly occurs as a respiratory compensation to metabolic acidosis caused by conditions like **diabetic ketoacidosis**
- **Apneustic breathing**

  Characterized by prolonged inspiratory spasm. Seen in mid pons lesion with vagus cut
- **Ondine's Curse**
  - Also called **congenital central hypoventilation syndrome**
  - Characterized by the loss of involuntary control of breathing during sleep

Chemical Regulation of Respiration

Chemicals like O_2, CO_2 and H^+ regulate respiration through chemoreceptors. There are two types of chemoreceptors: central chemoreceptors and peripheral chemoreceptors.

Central Chemoreceptors

- Central chemoreceptors are present in ventral surface of medulla.
- They are more sensitive to increase in arterial PCO_2.
- Central chemoreceptors monitor the H^+ concentration of cerebrospinal fluid (CSF). **Central chemoreceptors are mainly stimulated by H^+ ions.**

Peripheral Chemoreceptors

- Peripheral chemoreceptors are in carotid bodies and aortic bodies.
- Carotid bodies are innervated by glossopharyngeal nerves (CN IX).
- Aortic bodies are innervated by vagus nerve (CN X).
- These nerve fibers are 2–5 μm in diameter and conduct at relatively low rate of 7–12 m/s.
- Two types of cells are seen in carotid and aortic bodies: Type I cells or Glomus cells and Type II cells.
- Glomus cells are stimulated mainly by hypoxia. They store the neurotransmitter **"Dopamine"**.
- Dopamine acts through D_2 receptor in type I cells.
- Whenever there is low PO_2 (hypoxia), O_2-sensitive K^+ channels in glomus cells close. Accumulation of K^+ inside the glomus cells leads to a state of depolarization. Such depolarization opens calcium channels leading to calcium influx. Influx

of calcium causes release of the neurotransmitter **dopamine** which stimulates the afferent nerve endings; and hypoxia signal is conveyed to brain.

Chemoreflex

- Chemoreflex is seen when chemoreceptors are activated.
- Hypoxia, hypercarbia and acidosis activate this reflex.
- Effect of this reflex—Hyperventilation

HYPOXIA AND ITS TYPES

- Hypoxia is defined as the deficiency of oxygen at the tissue level.
- Usually, the brain is affected first in hypoxia where it causes loss of consciousness in 10–20 seconds and death in 4–5 minutes.

There are four important types of hypoxia: hypoxic hypoxia, anemic hypoxia, stagnant hypoxia and histotoxic hypoxia

1. Hypoxic hypoxia
- Characterized by low tissue and arterial PO_2
- **Causes:** High altitude, COPD
- Since arterial PO_2 is less, peripheral chemoreceptors are stimulated in hypoxic hypoxia
- **Cyanosis:** Bluish discoloration of skin, when the concentration of reduced hemoglobin in capillary blood exceeds 40 g/L (4 g/dL), is seen in hypoxic hypoxia
- Oxygen therapy with 100% pure oxygen is very helpful in this type of hypoxia

2. Anemic hypoxia
- Characterized by reduction in hemoglobin concentration and reduced oxygen content in blood
- Arterial PO_2 is normal-peripheral chemoreceptors are NOT stimulated
- Anemic hypoxia is seen in carbon monoxide poisoning. Hyperbaric oxygen therapy is helpful in treatment

3. Stagnant hypoxia
- Also called ischemic hypoxia or circulatory hypoxia or hypoperfusion hypoxia
- Arteriovenous O_2 difference (a-v-O_2 difference) is increased in stagnant hypoxia
- Commonly seen in congestive cardiac failure
- Cyanosis is present

4. Histotoxic hypoxia
- Occurs due to blockage of cellular enzymes that utilize oxygen
- Commonly seen in cyanide poisoning
- Cyanide inhibits cytochrome oxidase enzyme in mitochondria leading to blockage of oxidative phosphorylation
- Arteriovenous O_2 difference (a-v-O_2 difference) is decreased in histotoxic hypoxia

ENVIRONMENTAL PHYSIOLOGY

High Altitude Physiology and Pathophysiology

- The most important problem associated with high altitude is "hypoxia". All the compensatory mechanisms develop to tackle this hypoxia effectively.
- Acclimatization refers to the changes in body tissues in response to long-term exposure to low PO_2.
- Physiological compensatory responses to high altitude hypoxia are:
  - **Increase in pulmonary ventilation:** Earliest response, Oxygen dissociation curve shifts to RIGHT.
  - **Increased numbers of red blood cells:** Erythropoietin increases RBC count and hemoglobin concentration.
  - **Increased vascularity of the peripheral tissues:** Vascular endothelial growth factor (VEGF)—promotes angiogenesis.
  - Increased diffusing capacity of the lungs.
  - Increased ability of the tissue cells to use O_2 despite low PO_2.

- **Acute mountain sickness (AMS)**
    - Develops 6–12 hours after ascent to a high altitude.
    - Characterized by nonspecific symptoms like headache and nausea.
    - Symptoms resolve spontaneously if the subject **descends to lower altitude.**
- **Chronic mountain sickness**
    - Also called **Monge's disease.**
    - Characterized by excessive erythrocytosis, pulmonary hypertension (moderate to severe), Cor pulmonale.
    - This condition is usually treated with venesection and acetazolamide.
- **High altitude pulmonary edema (HAPE)**
    - Lung responds to hypoxia by vasoconstriction. HAPE develops within 2–4 days after arrival at high altitude.
    - Treatment involves Immediate descent to lower altitude, administration of oxygen (4–6 L/min) and calcium channel blocker nifedipine.
- **High altitude cerebral edema (HACE)**
    - HACE is considered the extreme form of AMS.
    - Treatment involves immediate descent to lower altitude, administration of oxygen (2–4 L/min) and dexamethasone.

Deep Sea Physiology and Pathophysiology

- Basic problem encountered during deep sea descent is high atmospheric pressure.
- Sea level pressure is 1 atm.
- At a depth of 10 m in sea, it becomes 2 atm (high).
- **Decompression sickness**
    - Also called Caisson's disease, Dysbarism, Diver's palsy.
    - Nitrogen gets decompressed and released out as bubbles.
    - **Nitrogen narcosis:** Nitrogen gas can easily cross the blood-brain barrier leading to euphoria, overconfidence, deterioration in judgment.
    - Pain in joints and muscles (bends), shortness of breath (chokes).
    - Air embolism.
    - Decompression sickness is treated by placing the victim in hyperbaric chamber and decreasing the pressure slowly so that gases come out slowly.

Space Physiology and Pathophysiology

Gravitational forces (G forces) are experienced by the body during flight and space travel. Such G forces include Positive G force and Negative G force.

Positive G

- When an individual is subjected to positive G, blood is pushed toward the lowermost part of the body.
- Features of positive G are venous pooling in lower limbs, decrease in cerebral pressure decreases, unconsciousness, low blood flow to blood vessels of eye leading to black out of vision.

Negative G

- When an individual is subjected to negative G, blood is pushed toward the head end.
- Features of negative G are increase in venous return and cerebral pressure, congestion of head and neck vessels, hyperemia of the eye leading to red out.

MUST KNOW

Exposure to microgravity in astronauts causes motion sickness, decrease in red blood cell mass, decrease in muscle strength, decrease in work capacity, loss of calcium and phosphate from the bones leading to loss of bone mass.

6. CARDIOVASCULAR PHYSIOLOGY

CARDIAC POTENTIALS

Two types of action potentials are seen in heart as follows:

1. **Pacemaker potential:** Mainly seen at SA node.
2. **Ventricular action potential:** Mainly seen in the ventricular myocardium.

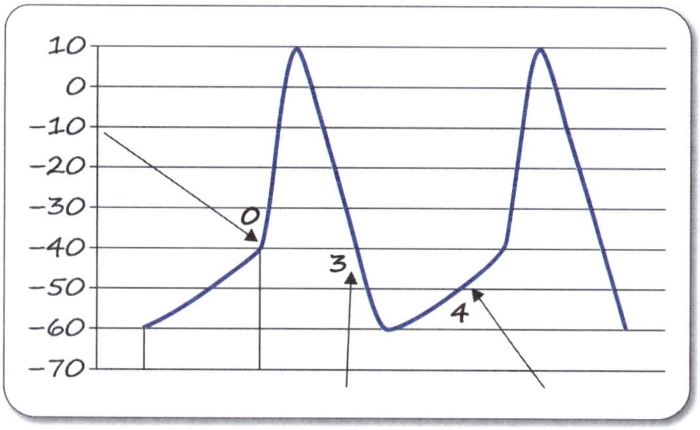

Pacemaker action potential

Phases	Ions responsible
Prepotential phase (corresponds to Phase 4 of ventricular action potential)	It oscillates between –60 mV and –40 mV Ions responsible: 1. Decline in potassium (K^+) current. 2. Funny currents (I_f). 3. Influx of calcium ions through T-type ("transient") calcium channels
Depolarization phase (corresponds to phase 0 of ventricular action potential)	Inward Ca^{++} currents through L-type calcium channels
Repolarization phase (corresponds to phase 3 of ventricular action potential)	Efflux of potassium ions

- **Sympathetic nervous system—Norepinephrine** increases heart rate by increasing the slope of prepotential phase.
- **Parasympathetic nervous system—Acetylcholine** decreases heart rate by decreasing the slope of prepotential phase.
- Funny currents are also called "Hyperpolarization-activated cyclic nucleotide–gated (HCN) channels." They are present in visual rods, cones, olfactory epithelium, SA Node. Funny current channel blocker—Ivabradine—is useful to reduce heart rate in sinus tachycardia.

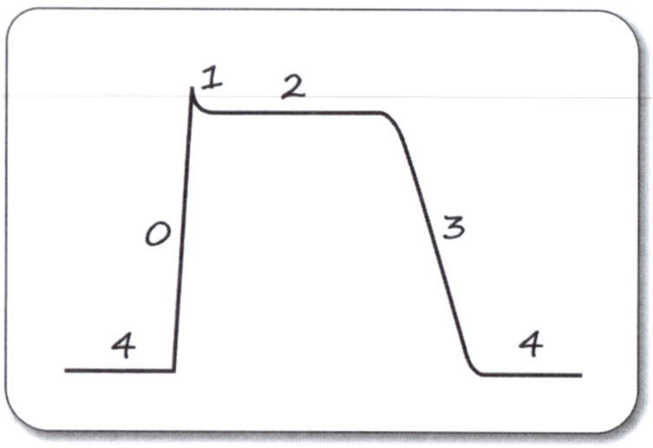

Ventricular action potential

Phases	Ions responsible
Phase 0—Rapid depolarization	Due to entry of sodium
Phase 1—Initial repolarization	Efflux of potassium ions
Phase 2—Plateau phase	Influx of calcium ions through (L-type) calcium channels
Phase 3—Late repolarization	Efflux of potassium ions
Phase 4—Return to resting Membrane Potential	By Na^+ K^+ ATPase

CONDUCTION SYSTEM OF HEART

SA node: "The Pacemaker"—Impulse originates here. Generates impulse at fastest rate (100 impulses/min)

AV node

- AV node conduction is slow. There is a delay of about 0.1 second in spread of impulse.
- This delay is mainly responsible for the sequential contraction of atrium followed by ventricles. It is for this reason AV node is also called **"Gatekeeper"** to the ventricles.
- Has the slowest impulse conduction velocity (0.04 m/s) due to less number of gap junctions.

Bundle of His: Receives the impulse from AV node

Purkinje fibers

- These are interconnected by numerous gap junctions.
- Have the fastest impulse conduction velocity (4 m/s).

Last parts of the heart to be depolarized are posterobasal portion of the left ventricle, the pulmonary conus, and the uppermost portion of the septum. These are the areas which repolarize first.

ELECTROCARDIOGRAM (ECG)

The ECG paper

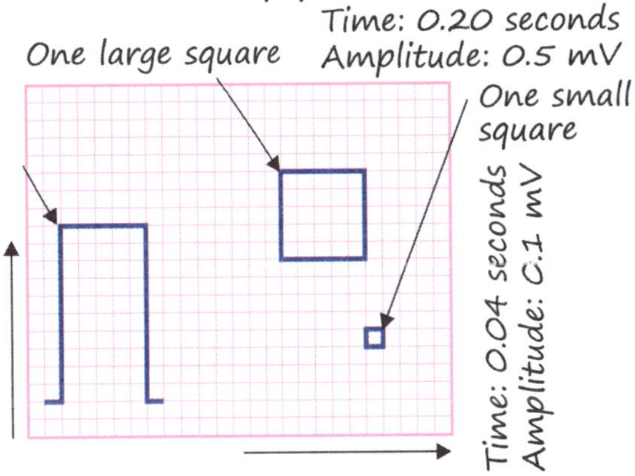

ECG waves

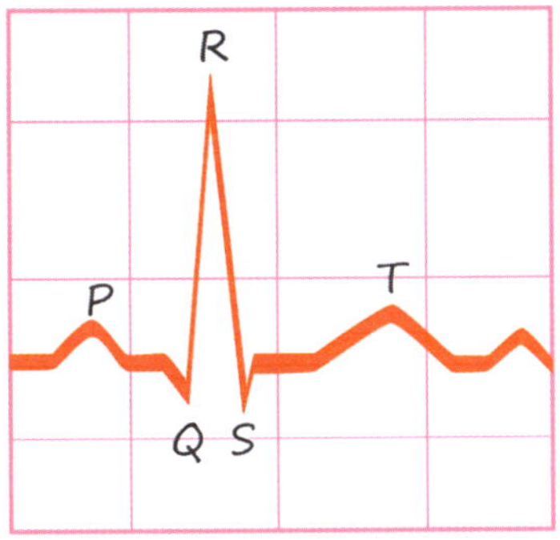

Wave	Cause
P wave	Atrial depolarization
QRS complex	Ventricular depolarization
T wave	Ventricular repolarization
U wave	Papillary muscle repolarization, Purkinje fiber repolarization

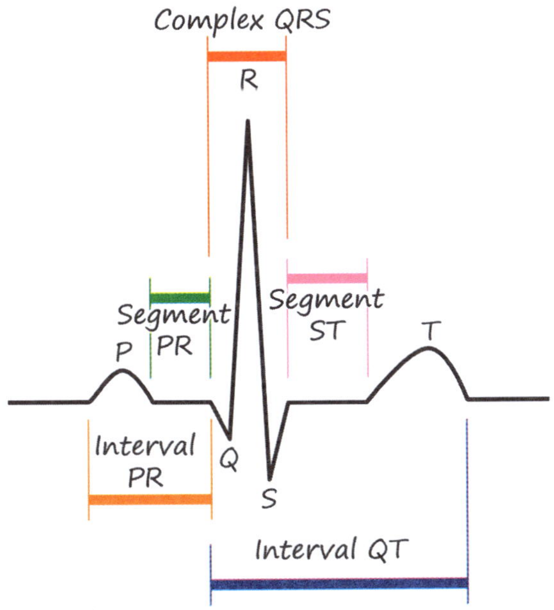

Segments	From to	Denotes
PR	From the end of P wave to the beginning of QRS complex	An isoelectric line that denotes the normal AV nodal delay
ST segment	From the end of S wave (J point) to the beginning of T wave	An isoelectric line that denotes the plateau phase of ventricular action potential

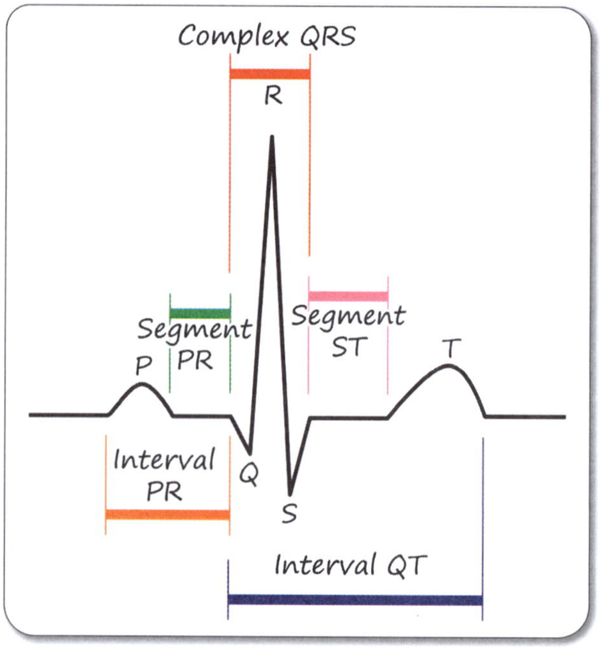

Intervals	From to	Normal value	Denotes
PR interval	From the onset of P wave to the beginning of QRS complex	0.12 to 0.20 sec	Atrioventricular (AV) conduction time
QT interval	From the onset of Q wave to the end of T wave	0.35 to 0.43 sec	Denotes ventricular depolarization and repolarization events
RR interval	Interval between two successive R waves	0.6–1 sec	Useful to calculate heart rate (HR). The formula is, HR = 1500/no. of small squares between two R waves

His Bundle Electrocardiogram (HBE)

- Usually done in patients with heart block.
- **His bundle electrocardiogram waves:** A wave (denotes AV node activation), H wave (denotes His bundle activation) and V wave (denotes ventricular depolarization).
- **His bundle electrocardiogram intervals:**
  - **PA interval:** From P wave in ECG to the A wave in HBE
  - **AH interval:** From A wave to the start of H wave
  - **HV interval:** From the start of H wave to the start of V wave

CARDIAC CYCLE

MUST KNOW

- **Duration of cardiac cycle:** 0.8 sec for a heart rate of 75 beats/min
- **Atrial systole:** 0.1 seconds
- **Atrial diastole:** 0.7 seconds
- **Ventricular systole:** 0.3 seconds
- **Ventricular diastole:** 0.5 seconds
- For a heart rate of 200 beats/min, duration of cardiac cycle is **0.3 seconds** (Systole - 0.14 seconds and

  Diastole – 0.16 sec). Fall in diastole duration is more during increased heart rates during exercise.

Ventricular Systole

- Comprises three sub phases, namely isovolumic contraction, rapid ejection phase and slow ejection phase.
- **First heart sound (S_1) occurs during isovolumic contraction.**
- **Rapid ejection phase:** Aortic and pulmonary valve are opened, ventricles eject blood rapidly.
- **Slow ejection phase:** Ventricular pressure starts decreasing and the ejection slowly falls.
- At the end of systole, still 50 mL of blood remains, which is called end systolic volume. **ESV = 50 mL**

Ventricular Diastole

- Comprises five sub phases namely protodiastole, isovolumic relaxation, rapid filling phase, slow filling phase and lastly filling due to atrial contraction.
- At the end of protodiastole, aortic and pulmonary valves close. This is responsible for **second heart sound (S_2).**
- Pressure inside the ventricles falls even more without any change in volume- isovolumic relaxation.
- Opening of AV valves leads to rapid filling of ventricles. This rapid inflow of blood vibrates ventricular walls and causes **third heart sound (S_3).**

- ***Slow filling phase is also called diastasis.***
- *Since ventricular filling is largely passive, only the last part of its filling is due to active atrial contraction (atrial kick). If the ventricle is not properly relaxing (stiff ventricle), atrium contracts forcefully to fill ventricles. This causes **fourth heart sound (S_4).***
- *At the end of diastole, the amount of blood present in ventricles is 120 mL, which is the end diastolic volume (EDV).*

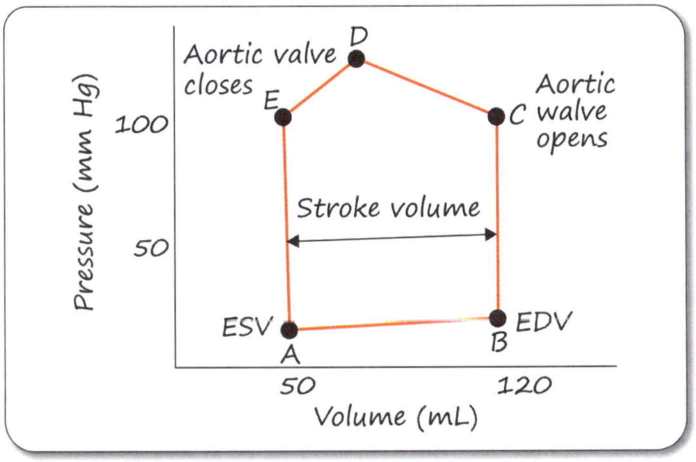

Ventricular pressure volume loop

- ***Point A—denotes mitral valve opening.***
- *Point B—denotes mitral valve closure. This causes first heart sound (S_1).*
- *ESV is 50 mL and EDV is 120 mL.*
- *At point E, aort ic valve closes. This causes second heart sound (S_2).*
- ***Stroke volume = End diastolic volume - End systolic volume.***
  Stroke volume = 120–50 = 70 mL
- *Ejection fraction= Stroke volume/End diastolic volume × 100 = 70/120 × 100. Ejection fraction normally is about 55–65%.*

Wiggers Diagram

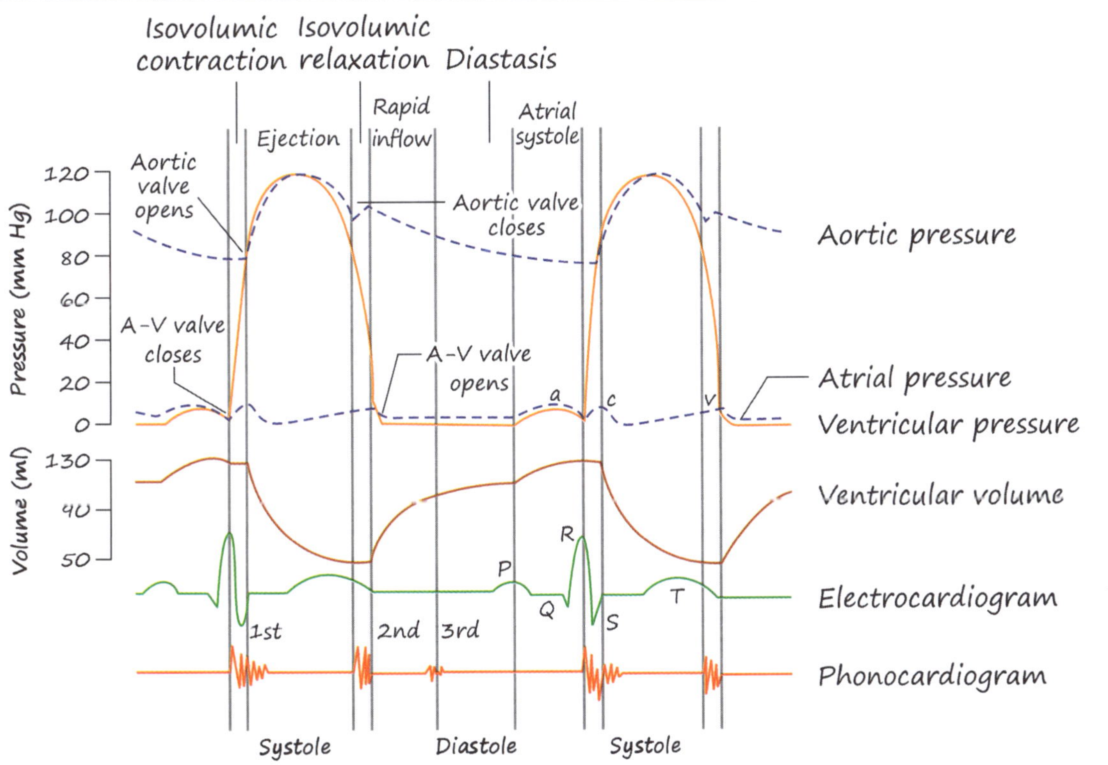

Heart sound	Correlates with
1st heart sound	R wave
2nd heart sound	End of T wave
3rd heart sound	Rapid filling phase
4th heart sound	P wave

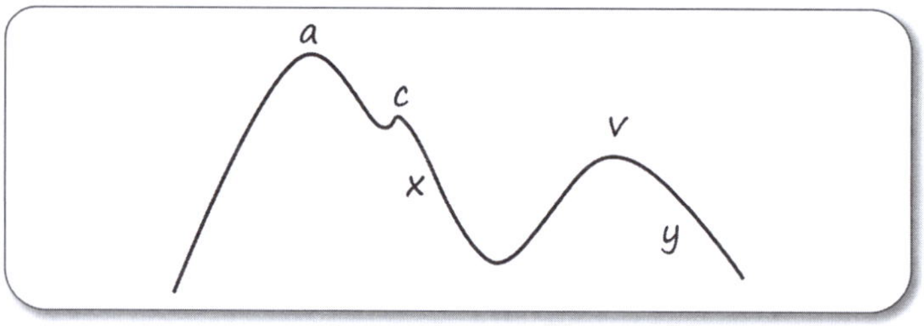

Jugular venous pressure waveform

JVP waveforms	Characteristics
"a" wave	Due to right atrial contraction (atrial systole)
"c" wave	Due to bulging of tricuspid valve into right atrium during isovolumic contraction
"x" descent	Denotes fall in right atrial pressure during atrial relaxation
"v" wave	Due to right atrial filling (atrial diastole)
"y" descent	Due to rapid emptying of right atrium once tricuspid valve opens

JVP abnormality	Cause(s)
Large "a" wave	Tricuspid stenosis, right atrial myxoma
Cannon "a" wave	Atrioventricular (AV) dissociation (complete heart block)
Absent "a" wave	Atrial fibrillation
Prominent "x" descent	Constrictive pericarditis
Blunted "x" descent	Tricuspid regurgitation
Tall "v" wave	Severe tricuspid regurgitation
Prominent "y" descent	Tricuspid regurgitation, constrictive pericarditis (Friedreich sign)
Blunted "y" descent	Tricuspid stenosis, right atrial myxoma

CARDIAC OUTPUT

- Cardiac output is the product of heart rate (HR) and stroke volume (SV).
- Normal cardiac output value for men is 5.6 L/min and that for women is 4.9 L/min.
- Cardiac index is expressing cardiac output per square meter of body surface area.
- Normal cardiac index for adults is 3.2 L/min/m^2 of body surface area.
- Cardiac output can be increased by increase in heart rate by **sympathetic activation.**
- Stroke volume is affected by three important factors namely, preload, afterload and myocardial contractility.

1. **Preload:**
    - Preload is the venous return which eventually comes to the left ventricle as end-diastolic volume.
    - Stroke volume is directly proportional to preload (end-diastolic volume).
    - Increase in preload increases cardiac output which can be explained by **Frank-Starling law.**
    - **Frank-Starling law** states that "the force of contraction of heart is directly proportional to the initial length of muscle fibers, before the onset of contraction".
    - Best marker for preload is end-diastolic volume.
2. **Myocardial Contractility**
    - Contractility of the cardiac muscle cells can only be increased by sympathetic nervous system activation (norepinephrine).
    - Increase in myocardial contractility increases cardiac output.
    - Best marker for myocardial contractility is ejection fraction.
3. **Afterload**
    - Afterload is the force against which ventricles must contract (aortic pressure) and eject the blood.
    - Afterload is inversely related to stroke volume. If aortic pressure rises, stroke volume decreases and cardiac output decreases.
    - Best markers for afterload are aortic pressure and total peripheral resistance.

MUST KNOW

- **Distribution of cardiac output and oxygen consumption of various body organs:**
    - Blood flow (mL/min) is highest for liver: 1500 mL/min
    - Blood flow (mL/100 g/min) is highest for kidney: 420 mL/100 g/min
    - Arteriovenous oxygen difference (mL/L) is highest for heart: 114 mL/L
    - Arteriovenous oxygen difference (mL/L) is lowest for kidney: 14 mL/L

Contd...

- O_2 consumption (mL/min) is highest for liver: 51 mL/min
- O_2 consumption (mL/100 g/min) is highest for heart: 10 mL/100 g/min
- Highest percentage of cardiac output that goes to liver: 27.8%
- Highest percentage of O_2 consumption is by liver: 20.4%

Measurement of cardiac output:

- Fick's method—gold standard method for measuring cardiac output
- Based on Fick's principle which states that "the amount of a substance taken up by an organ per unit of time is equal to the arterial level of the substance minus the venous level (A-V difference) times the blood flow".

$$\text{So, Cardiac output} = \frac{O_2 \text{ consumed in mL/min}}{\text{Arteriovenous oxygen difference}}$$

- Other methods for estimating cardiac output are indicator (dye) dilution method, and thermodilution method.

CORONARY CIRCULATION

- Has a very high basal oxygen consumption (8 -10 mL O2/min/100 g).
- The highest A-V O_2 difference of a major organ is 10-13 mL/100 mL.
- Normal Coronary blood flow: 60-80 mL/100 g/min or 250 mL/min viz. 5% of resting cardiac output.
- The peak left coronary flow occurs at the end of isovolumetric relaxation (diastole).
- Local metabolism is the primary controller of coronary flow—O_2 demand is a major factor.
- Local accumulation of adenosine and nitric oxide increases coronary blood flow.
- Major role of coronary circulation is to provide myocardium with oxygen and further myocardial oxygen consumption.
- Primary determinants of myocardial oxygen consumption are:
  - Intramyocardial tension
  - Contractile state of the myocardium
  - Heart rate
  - Duration of Systole

VASCULAR PHYSIOLOGY

Hematopoiesis

Age	Site of Hematopoiesis
3 weeks–3 months	Yolk sac
3–5 months	Liver, spleen
5–9 months	Red bone marrow in long and flat bones
After birth till 20 years of age	Red bone marrow in long and flat bones
>20 years	Only in flat bones like ilia

Erythropoiesis—Formation of Red Blood Cells

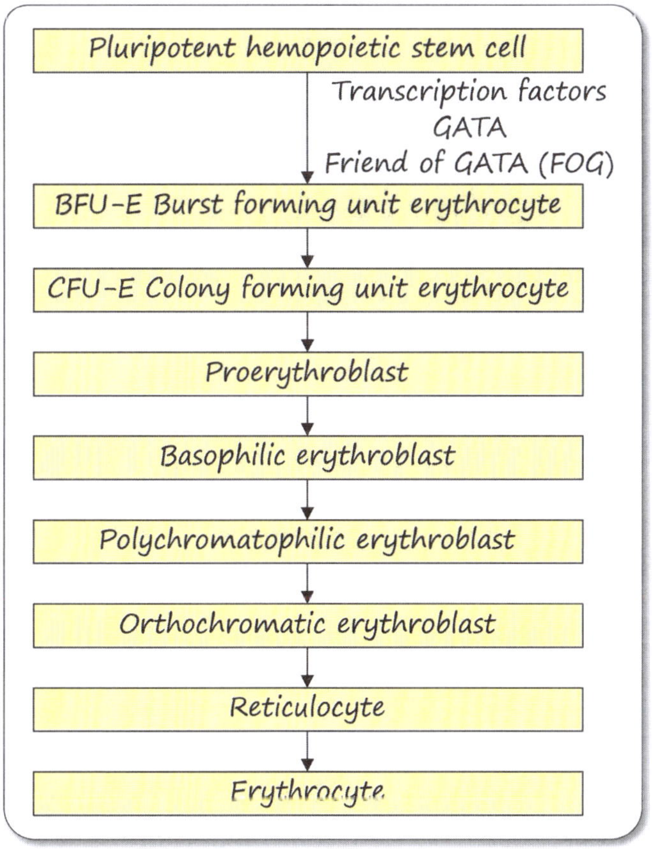

- Erythroid burst forming unit (BFU-E)—earliest committed erythroid progenitor cells
- Colony forming unit-erythrocytes (CFU-E)—has got the highest number of erythropoietin receptors
- Basophilic erythroblast—synthesis of hemoglobin starts in this stage
- Polychromatophilic erythroblast—hemoglobin appears
- Orthochromatic (late) erythroblast—full complement of hemoglobin

Contd...

- Reticulocyte—immature RBCs without a nucleus, ribosomal RNA stained by supravital stains
- Erythrocyte—size is 7.2 μ diameter, Biconcave disc shaped
- Erythropoietin (EPO):
  - Major factor regulating red cell production
  - Kidney is the major source
  - Major stimulus for secretion of EPO is "Hypoxia"
  - Receptor for erythropoietin—Cytokine receptor that activates JAK/STAT signaling cascade
  - The transcription factor that up regulates erythropoietin synthesis is called hypoxia-inducible factor (HIF)-lα
  - Recombinant human erythropoietin (rHuEPO) drugs—Epoetin alfa, Darbepoetin alfa

Leukopoiesis—Formation of White Blood Cells

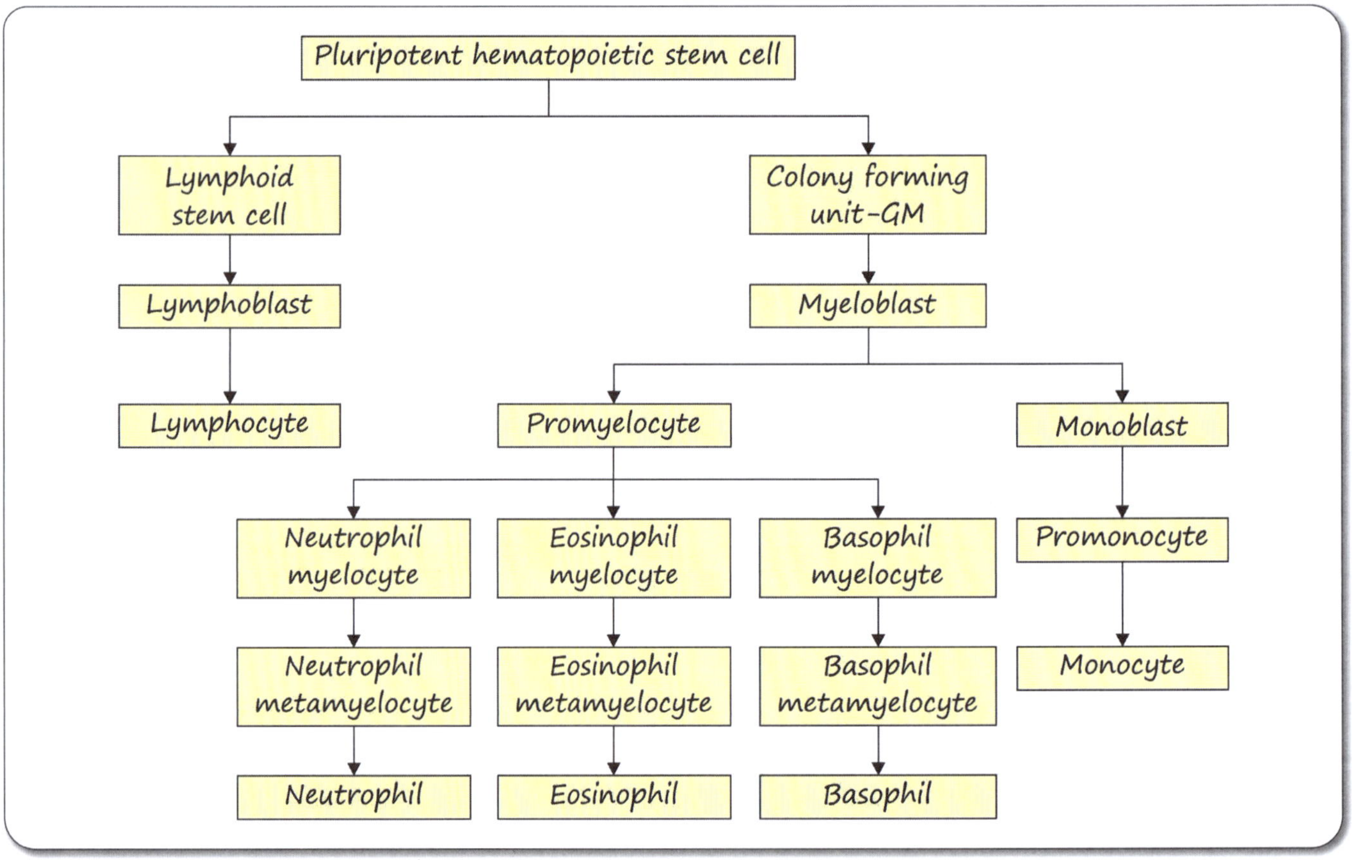

- Important factors that regulate Leukopoiesis are: Granulocyte-monocyte colony-stimulating factor (GMCSF), Granulocyte colony-stimulating factor (G-CSF)
- Filgrastim—recombinant human G-CSF
- Sargramostim—recombinant human GM-CSF
- Pegfilgrastim—conjugation product of filgrastim
- Lenograstim—glycosylated form of recombinant G-CSF
- These drugs are useful in Cancer Chemotherapy-Induced Neutropenia
- Interleukin 5—for eosinophil development
- Interleukin 3, 4—for basophil development

Thrombopoiesis—Formation of Platelets

Pluripotent hematopoietic stem cell
↓
GM-CSF thrombo
↓
Megakaryocyte
↓
Platelets

- Important factors that regulate thrombopoiesis are called as megakaryocyte growth factors. They are Thrombopoietin (TPO), IL-11
- **Oprelvekin—recombinant form of IL-11:** Commonly used in cancer chemotherapy induced thrombocytopenia
- **Romiplostim—Thrombopoietin agonist:** Useful in treatment of chronic immune thrombocytopenia
- **Eltrombopag—Thrombopoietin agonist:** Useful in treatment of chronic immune thrombocytopenia, thrombocytopenia in hepatitis C

BLOOD GROUPS AND THEIR CHARACTERISTICS

Blood group	Characteristics
ABO blood group system	• Inheritance of ABO blood groups—"Autosomal codominant" • ABO blood group antigens are present in blood, saliva, semen, amniotic fluid • O group—Universal donors • AB group—Universal recipients
The Rh system	• Second most important blood group system • D antigen is most important • Rh incompatibility—"Hemolytic disease of the fetus and newborn" or Erythroblastosis fetalis: damage basal ganglia leading to kernicterus
The P system	• Autoantibodies to P is called Donath-Landsteiner antibodies which leads to paroxysmal cold hemoglobinuria—seen in syphilis • P antigen serves as cellular receptor for parvovirus B19 and E. coli
The Kell system	• Absence of kell system leads to **McLeod phenotype** characterized by RBCs with spines (Acanthocytes), Cardiac defects
The Duffy system	• Duffy antigens are the receptor for malaria causing **Plasmodium vivax** • If Duffy antigen receptor for cytokines (DARC) is absent—it leads to mild neutropenia

CHARACTERISTICS OF BLOOD VESSELS

Vessel	Cross-sectional area (m^2)	Blood flow velocity	% of blood contained
Aorta	4.5 (min)	40 cm/s (max)	2
Artery	20		8
Arteriole	400		1
Capillary	4500 (max)	0.05 cm/s (min)	5
Venule	4000		
Vein	40	20 cm/s	54 (max)
Vena cava	18		

Starling Forces at Capillary

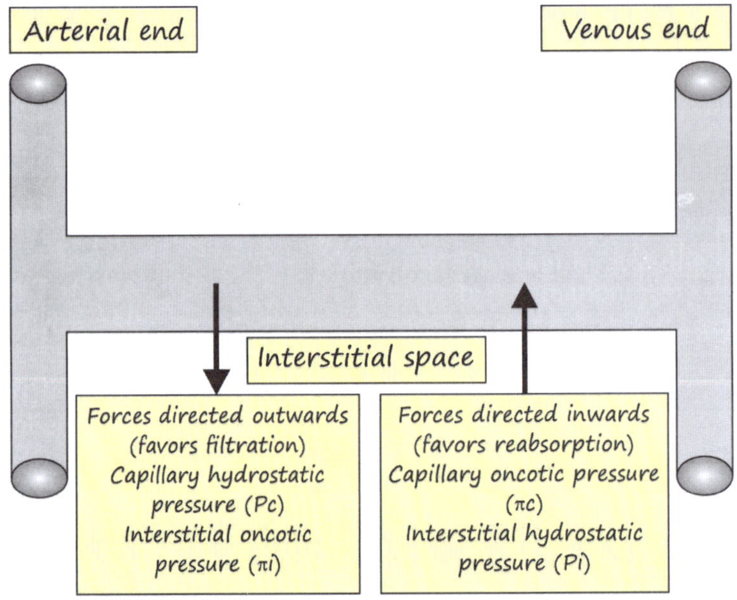

- Net filtering force = Forces favoring filtration—Forces favoring reabsorption
- Net filtering force = $(Pc + \pi i) - (\pi c + Pi)$

MUST KNOW

Important Points about Blood Vessels

Vessel With

- Maximum cross-sectional area: Capillaries
- Minimum cross-sectional area: Aorta
- Maximum blood flow velocity: Aorta
- Minimum blood flow velocity: Capillaries
- Maximum diameter: Vena cava
- Maximum % of blood stored: Veins
- Resistance vessels: Arterioles
- Capacitance vessels: Veins
- Exchange vessels: Capillaries
- Windkessel vessel: Aorta
- Temperature regulation: AV shunts
- Maximum smooth muscle content: Arterioles

HEMODYNAMICS

- Factors determining blood flow are expressed by the Poiseuille-Hagen formula as follows:

$$F = (P_A - P_B) * \pi r^4/8\ \eta L$$

- In this formula: Pressure difference $(P_A - P_B)$, Radius of the vessel (r^4), Viscosity of the fluid (η), Length of the vessel (L).
- If the radius of blood vessels is halved because of stenosis, blood flow will be reduced by 16 times.
- **Fahraeus-Lindqvist effect:** This effect is seen mainly in capillaries where RBCs flow in the center which leaves cell free plasma near the vessel wall.
- Resistance and blood flow are always inversely related. The relationship between them is called **"Fourth power law."** This means that if the radius of the vessel wall decreases from 4 cm to 2 cm, the resistance increases by 16 times.
- Blood flow inside the vessel can be laminar flow or streamlined flow (without noise) and turbulent flow (with noise).
- Whether the blood flow is laminar or turbulent is determined by Reynolds number.
- Reynolds number (Re) = $\rho DV/\eta$, Where, ρ -density of the fluid, D—diameter of the tube, V—velocity, η—Viscosity
- If Re <2000, flow is laminar; if Re >3000, flow is turbulent; and if Re is between 2000 and 3000, flow is transitional.

BLOOD COAGULATION

Clotting factors

Factor	Name	Deficiency leads to
I	Fibrinogen	Afibrinogenemia
II	Prothrombin	Hypoprothrombinemia (Hemorrhagic tendency in liver disease)
III	Thromboplastin	
IV	Calcium	
V	Proaccelerin, labile factor,	Parahemophilia
VII	Proconvertin, stable factor	Hypoconvertinemia
VIII	Antihemophilic factor (AHF), antihemophilic factor A	Hemophilia A (classic hemophilia)
IX	Plasma thromboplastic component (PTC), Christmas factor, antihemophilic factor B	Hemophilia B (Christmas disease)
X	Stuart-Prower factor	Stuart-Prower factor deficiency
XI	Plasma thromboplastin antecedent (PTA), antihemophilic factor C	PTA deficiency
XII	Hageman factor, glass factor	Hageman trait
XIII	Fibrin-stabilizing factor, Laki-Lorand factor	Abnormal Clot Solubility

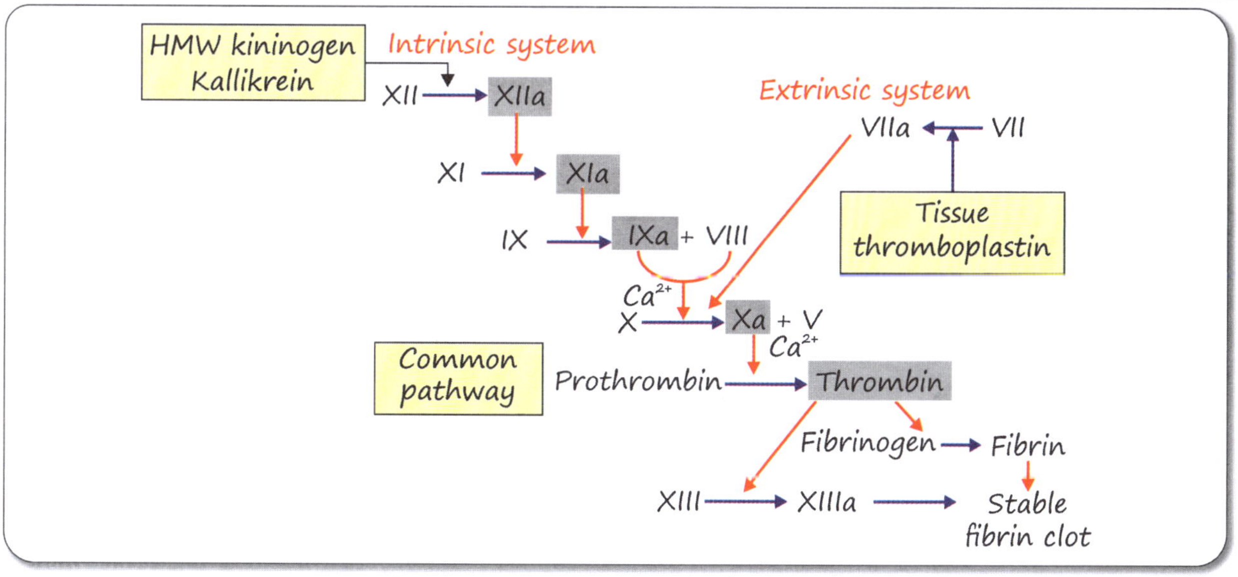

Blood coagulation

- Factors of intrinsic pathway: XII, XI, IX, VIII
- Factors of extrinsic pathway: factor III, factor VII
- Factors of common pathway: X, I, II, IV, V, XIII
- Activated Partial Thromboplastin Time (APTT): Measures Intrinsic and common pathways. Normal value: 26-40 seconds
- Prothrombin Time (PT): Measures Extrinsic and common pathways. Normal value: 11-16 seconds
- Antithrombin III and heparin inactivates factors IX, X, XI, XII
- Thrombin Thrombomodulin complex inactivates factors Va, VIIIa
- Vitamin K-Dependent Factors: Factor II, Factor VII, Factor IX, Factor X, protein C and protein S
- Warfarin: Anticoagulant-antagonist of vitamin K

BLOOD PRESSURE

- Blood pressure is defined as "the lateral pressure exerted by the column of blood on wall of arteries".
- Blood pressure is the product of cardiac output and total peripheral resistance.
- **Systolic blood pressure (SBP)**: 120 mm Hg, **Diastolic blood pressure (DBP)**: 80 mm Hg
- Difference between the systolic and diastolic pressures (SBP – DBP) is pulse pressure.
- Mean arterial blood pressure = Diastolic pressure + 1/3 of pulse pressure
- Normal mean arterial pressure is around 93–100 mm Hg.
- Velocity of blood flow (kinetic energy) and the pressure (potential energy) is interrelated by the Bernoulli's principle which is "the sum of the kinetic energy of flow and the potential energy—is constant".

MUST KNOW

Various Types of Pressures to Remember

	Systole	Diastole
Right Atrium	5 mm Hg	0
Right Ventricle	15–30 mm Hg	0–5 mm Hg
Pulmonary Artery	15–30 mm Hg	10 mm Hg
Left Atrium	12 mm Hg	4 mm Hg
Left Ventricle	90–140 mm Hg	4–12 mm Hg
Aorta	90–140 mm Hg	60–90 mm Hg

Regulation of Blood Pressure

Two modes of regulating BP are nervous regulation (short term regulation) and chemical regulation.

Short-term regulation of BP

- Baroreflex
- Chemoreflex
- CNS ischemic response

Intermediate-term regulation of BP

- Capillary fluid shift
- Stress relaxation

Long-term regulation of BP

- Renin angiotensin aldosterone system (RAAS)
- Regulation of blood volume by kidney

Nervous Regulation (Short Term Regulation)

Baroreflex

- Mediated by sensors which are the stretch receptors known as baroreceptors, which are Carotid sinus—a small dilation in internal carotid artery and Aortic arch—in the aortic arch wall.
- Carotid sinus is innervated by the branch of glossopharyngeal nerve called "**carotid sinus nerve**". It is also called "**Herring's nerve**".
- Aortic arch is innervated by branch of the vagus nerve called "**aortic depressor nerve**". It is also called "**Cyon's nerve**".
- Nerves that innervates baroreceptors are collectively called **"Buffer nerves"** because they neutralize changes in BP.
- Whenever blood pressure increases, baroreceptors increase their discharge and send their impulse to medulla which ultimately decreases the blood pressure. Baroreflex is a classic example of **negative feedback mechanism.**

Baroreflex mechanism

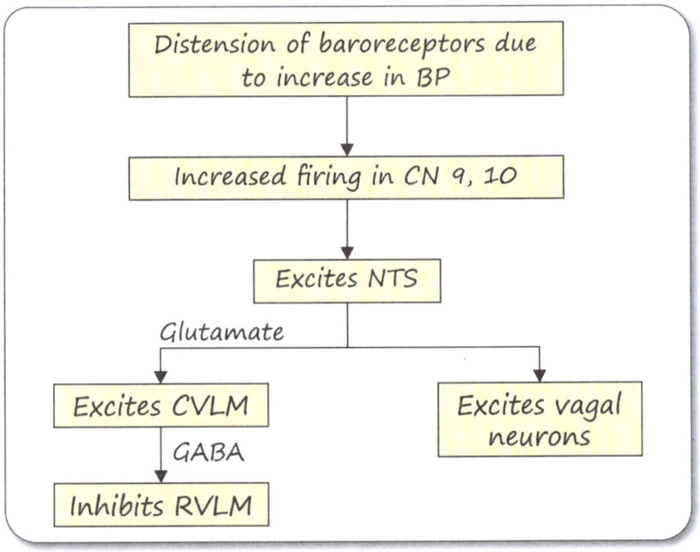

- Center for baroreflex—Nucleus Tractus Solitarius (NTS).
- Rostral ventrolateral medulla (RVLM) is the sympathetic center.
- In simple terms, "increased baroreceptor discharge inhibits the tonic discharge of sympathetic nerves and excites the vagal innervation of the heart".
- Carotid sinus massage (Czermak-Hering test): Baroreceptors activated—vagal parasympathetic fibers decrease the heart rate. Useful to reduce heart rate in supraventricular tachycardia.
- Baroreceptors—regulates BP in the range of 70–150 mm Hg.

Chemoreflex

Chemoreceptors—Regulates BP in the range of 40–70 mm Hg.

CNS Ischemic Response

- Whenever mean arterial pressure falls below 40 mm Hg, there is marked BP rise as high as 250 mm Hg.
- It is also called the "last-ditch stand" pressure control mechanism.

Mayer waves

Oscillations of the above said nervous pressure control mechanisms are usually seen in the form of waves. Such waves are called **"Vasomotor waves" or "Mayer waves".**

Traube–Hering waves

- Traube–Hering waves are the fluctuations in blood pressure synchronized with respiration.
- Normally during inspiration, systolic blood pressure decreases ≤10 mm Hg and there is increase in arterial pressure during the early part of expiration.

Chemical Regulation of Blood Pressure

Vasoconstrictors (Increase BP)

- **Urotensin-II:** Most potent
- Endothelin
  - Endothelin receptors are of two types, termed ET_A and ET_B
  - ET_A receptor—in vascular smooth muscle-mediates vasoconstriction and increases BP.
  - Endothelin receptor blocker Bosentan-useful in treatment of **pulmonary arterial hypertension.**
- Vasopressin
  - Vasopressin causes vasoconstriction by acting on its vascular V_1 receptor.
  - Vasopressin and its analog **Terlipressin** are useful in treatment of variceal bleeding.
- **Angiotensin II:** Constricts arteriolar smooth muscle leading to vasoconstriction and increase in BP.
- Norepinephrine

Vasodilators (Decrease BP)

- **Calcitonin gene-related peptide (CGRP):** Most potent vasodilator
- Nitric oxide
  - Also called **endothelium-derived relaxing factor (EDRF).**
  - Nitric oxide is synthesized from arginine. The enzyme responsible for its synthesis is nitric oxide synthase (NOS).
  - Nitric oxide acts by increasing the levels of second messenger cGMP.
  - Drugs like sildenafil that potentiate the actions of NO by inhibiting the phosphodiesterase enzymes that degrade cGMP—useful in treatment of erectile dysfunction
- Prostacyclins (PGI_2)
- Kinins
- Histamine

MUST KNOW

Important cardiac reflexes

- **Bainbridge reflex or atrial reflex**
  - This reflex is activated whenever there is increase in venous return to the heart.
  - Stimulation of SA node—increase heart rate **(Tachycardia).**
- **Bezold-Jarisch reflex**
  - Intracardiac injections of chemicals like serotonin, veratridine, capsaicin, phenylbiguanide activate this reflex.
  - The reflex responses are:
    - Apnea followed by rapid breathing
    - Hypotension
    - Bradycardia
  - This reflex is responsible for sinus bradycardia seen during myocardial infarction.

Contd...

- ***Cushing reflex***
  - *Cushing reflex is characterized by increase in BP and reflex decrease in heart rate (bradycardia).*
  - *It is mainly seen in conditions causing increase in intracranial pressure.*
- ***The Oculocardiac reflex***
  - *Also called* ***Aschner phenomenon or Aschner-Dagnini reflex.***
  - *This reflex is activated during traction applied to extraocular muscles and/or compression of the eyeball.*
  - *Afferents for this reflex travel through long and short ciliary nerves to the trigeminal nucleus.*
  - *Efferent travel through vagus nerve to the heart.*
  - *Oculocardiac reflex is characterized by* ***profound bradycardia.***
- ***Marey's Law***
  - *This law states that heart rate and BP are inversely related.*
  - *This law explains reflex bradycardia associated with increase in BP.*

Notes

7. ENDOCRINE PHYSIOLOGY

ENDOCRINE SYSTEM

- Major function of endocrine system is to maintain whole body homeostasis.
- The secretions of endocrine glands are usually the "**hormones**".
- **Secretin was the first hormone discovered by Bayliss and Starling.**
- Endocrine hormone secretion follows a typical negative feedback principle.
- Hypothalamus secretes releasing factor which stimulates the secretion of trophic factors from anterior pituitary. Trophic factors from anterior pituitary reach the target glands and stimulate the secretion of peripheral hormones which, as a part of feedback loop, inhibit both hypothalamic and pituitary hormones.

MUST KNOW

Two good examples can be cited where hormones are released in positive feedback manner. They are **Luteinizing Hormone (LH) Surge and Parturition**–plasma oxytocin level rises and causes further uterine contraction ultimately leading to the delivery of fetus. The name of this positive feedback reflex seen during parturition is called **FERGUSON REFLEX.**

CLASSIFICATION OF HORMONES

- Hormones are classified into four types follows:
  1. **Amino acid derivatives:** Tyrosine derivatives–Epinephrine, Norepinephrine, Dopamine, Thyroid hormones
  2. **Large protein hormones:** Insulin (51 amino acids), **Parathormone** (84 amino acids)
  3. **Steroid hormones:** Derivatives of cholesterol. synthesized in the smooth endoplasmic reticulum. Examples—Androgen, Estrogen, Aldosterone, Cortisol
  4. **Vitamin hormones:** Vitamin A and Vitamin D

ROLE OF HYPOTHALAMUS

Hypothalamic Releasing Hormones

Hypothalamic hormone	Role in anterior pituitary
Thyrotropin-releasing hormone (TRH)	Releases Thyrotropin (TSH), prolactin (PRL)
Corticotropin-releasing hormone (CRH)	Releases Adrenocorticotropin (ACTH), β-lipotropin
Gonadotropin-releasing hormone (GnRH)	Releases Luteinizing hormone (LH), Follicle-stimulating hormone (FSH)
Growth hormone-releasing hormone (GHRH)	Releases growth hormone

Contd...

Hypothalamic Inhibiting Hormones

Hypothalamic hormone	Role in anterior pituitary
Prolactin release-inhibiting hormone (PIH), "**Dopamine**"	Inhibits the release of prolactin
Growth hormone release-inhibiting hormone or "**Somatostatin**"	Inhibits the release of growth hormone

PITUITARY GLAND

- Pituitary gland is called the "**master gland**", it controls all the other major endocrine glands.
- Has two important components: Adenohypophysis or anterior pituitary and Neurohypophysis or posterior pituitary or pars nervosa

Anterior pituitary: five important cell types that secrete six important hormones, which are as follows:

1. Somatotrope- Growth hormone: Percentage of Total Secretory Cells (50%): maximum
2. Lactotrope- Prolactin
3. Gonadotrope- Follicle-stimulating hormone (FSH), Luteinizing hormone (LH)
4. Thyrotrope- Thyroid-stimulating hormone (TSH)
5. Corticotrope- Adrenocorticotropic hormone (ACTH)

- Somatotrope and lactotrope are acidophilic cells.
- Gonadotrope, thyrotrope and corticotrope are basophilic cells.

Growth Hormone

- Growth hormone (GH) is the most abundant anterior pituitary hormone.
- GH level markedly decreases with aging.
- Growth hormone is similar to prolactin: Their actions overlap.

Actions of Growth Hormone

- Classified as direct actions and indirect actions.
- Direct actions are due to growth hormone itself.
- Indirect action is mediated by somatomedins: Growth hormone acts in liver to produce certain substances called somatomedins. Somatomedins are also called Insulin-like growth factors (IGFs).
- Actions in bone are BOTH direct and indirect actions.

1. **Direct actions:**
   - Growth hormone stimulates the differentiation and proliferation of cartilage cells (chondrocytes) in the epiphyseal end plates of long bones.
   - Increases blood glucose
   - Promotes lipolysis
   - Increases protein synthesis
2. **Indirect actions:**
   - Insulin-like growth factor -1 (IGF-1) profoundly influences bone and cartilage growth
   - Antilipolytic

Factors that Increase Growth Hormone

- **Hypoglycemia**: Growth hormone is a "**diabetogenic hormone**". It increases blood glucose levels.
- **Anything that causes hypoglycemia like fasting, starvation, exercise, stress**
- During sleep – Particularly deep sleep (NREM stages 3 and 4)
- Protein rich meal
- Glucagon
- Free fatty acids
- REM sleep
- **Growth hormone receptor**: Cytokine receptor superfamily- Janus kinus JAK-STAT signaling pathway: Growth hormone receptor antagonist drug is Pegvisomant- useful in treatment of acromegaly (Growth hormone excess).

Factors that Decrease Growth Hormone

- Infusion of glucose: Failure of GH suppression after oral glucose load is a definitive diagnostic test for acromegaly
- Growth hormone release-inhibiting hormone or "Somatostatin"
- Cortisol

MUST KNOW

Pathologic Conditions Involving Growth Hormone

- Deficiency of growth hormone causes dwarfism.
- Excess levels of growth hormone cause **Gigantism** (before the closure of epiphysis) and **Acromegaly (After the closure of epiphysis).**
- **Laron dwarfism:**
  - Also called "growth hormone insensitivity syndrome".
  - Growth hormone levels are normal but there is resistance to growth hormone action due to problem in growth hormone receptor.
  - This condition is diagnosed by low IGF-I levels.
  - Treatment: recombinant human IGF-I namely **Mecasermin.**
- **Acromegaly**
  - GH hypersecretion: Due to the GH secreting somatotrope adenoma in anterior pituitary
  - Clinical features of acromegaly are bony overgrowth leading to frontal bossing, prognathism (mandibular enlargement), increased heel pad thickness (due to soft tissue overgrowth), sleep apnea (upper airway obstruction), Carpal tunnel syndrome, diabetes mellitus (GH is a hyperglycemic hormone).
  - **Treatment of acromegaly**
    - Surgical treatment like **Trans-sphenoidal surgical resection** of the microadenoma is the preferred treatment
    - Somatostatin analogue drugs like octreotide
    - Growth hormone receptor antagonist – Pegvisomant

PROLACTIN

- Prolactin is secreted from acidophilic Lactotropes in anterior pituitary.
- Hypothalamus inhibits prolactin secretion through Dopamine (D_2 receptor).

- Glucocorticoids and thyroid hormones inhibit prolactin secretion.
- Prolactin also acts through cytokine receptor family: Janus Kinase JAK – STAT pathway
- Prolactin produces milk.
- Prolactin inhibits GnRH secretion leading to decrease in levels of FSH and LH: Prolactin is the hormone responsible for lactational amenorrhea.
- In men, low level of Luteinizing Hormone (LH) due to prolactin leads to low testosterone levels, decreased spermatogenesis and loss of libido.
- Factors that increase prolactin level:
  - Marked increase in levels is seen during pregnancy and lactation
  - Suckling of nipples
  - Sexual intercourse
  - REM sleep
  - Exercise
- Factors that decrease prolactin level: Dopamine agonists like Bromocriptine, Somatostatin, Glucocorticoids and Thyroid hormones.

THYROID GLAND

Major hormones produced by thyroid gland are Triiodothyronine (T3), Tetraiodothyronine (T4) and Calcitonin—from Parafollicular C cells of thyroid gland.

Steps involved in the Synthesis of Thyroid Hormones

1. **Uptake of iodide (Iodine trapping)**
   - Iodine is the essential mineral required for thyroid hormone synthesis.
   - Iodide uptake is mediated by Sodium Iodide symporter (NIS).
   - **Sodium Iodide symporter (NIS)** is present in thyroid follicular cells, salivary glands, lactating breast, gastric mucosa, placenta. This channel protein is capable of concentrating iodide 20–40 times inside thyroid follicular cell (iodide trap).
   - Large amounts of iodide transiently inhibit thyroid iodide organification. This effect is called **Wolff–Chaikoff effect.**
   - Another iodine transporter, called **Pendrin,** is present in the apical side of thyroid follicular cell.
   - Pendrin is an iodide-chloride antiport that mediates iodide efflux to the lumen of follicular cell. It is also present in inner ear. Mutation in pendrin gene leads to Pendred syndrome characterized by goiter and sensorineural deafness.
2. **Synthesis and secretion of thyroglobulin**
   - Thyroglobulin is the protein precursor of thyroid hormones. It is a large glycoprotein.
   - Auto antibodies directed against thyroglobulin —anti-thyroglobulin antibodies (ATAs) are commonly seen in Hashimoto's thyroiditis.
3. **Oxidation of iodine**
   - Oxidation of iodide and its further reactions with the secreted thyroglobulin are mediated by an enzyme called "**thyroid peroxidase**".
   - **Thyroid peroxidase** is blocked by antithyroid drugs namely **Propylthiouracil, methimazole and carbimazole.**
4. **Coupling reaction**
   - Once iodide is oxidized, it is incorporated into tyrosine residues of thyroglobulin. This is called **organification** of iodine.
   - The first product is called monoiodotyrosine (MIT). MIT is further iodinated to form diiodotyrosine (DIT).
   - Two molecules of DIT condense to form the thyroid hormone **thyroxine (T_4).**
   - One molecule of monoiodotyrosine (MIT) couples with one molecule of diiodotyrosine (DIT) to form **triiodothyronine (T_3).**
   - Condensation of DIT with MIT forms small amount of **reverse T_3 (RT_3).**
5. **Storage of thyroid hormones:** Stored in the lumen of the follicle in the form of "**colloid**". This storage form of thyroid hormones (colloid) is sufficient to supply thyroid hormones for **2–3 months.**
6. **Release of thyroid hormones**
   - Colloid fused with the lysosomes which contains **proteases** that digest the thyroglobulin molecule and releases free T_3, T_4 and reverse T_3, MIT and DIT.
   - MIT and DIT are acted upon by an enzyme called "**Deiodinase**", that removes iodine from them and the iodine is **recycled** for further hormone synthesis.
   - **Deiodinase:** Contains a rare amino acid "**selenocysteine**" responsible for their enzymatic activity. Selenocysteine is the 21st amino acid in humans.

MUST KNOW

Thyroid Hormone Binding Proteins

- Once released into the blood, thyroid hormones bind with three important proteins as follows:
  1. Albumin
  2. Thyroxine-binding globulin (TBG): Major one: **highest affinity** for thyroid hormone binding
  3. Transthyretin (also called thyroxine-binding prealbumin)—it is the major thyroid hormone—binding protein in the cerebrospinal fluid.

Differences between thyroid hormones Thyroxine (T_4) Vs Triiodothyronine (T_3)	
T_3	T_4
It is more potent.	It is less potent.
Considered the active form.	Considered the precursor of T_3.
Half-life is 1 day (less).	Half-life is 7 days (more).
Only 20% of T_3 come from thyroid. Remaining 80% is from peripheral conversion of T_4.	80% of T_4 comes from thyroid gland.
Plasma protein binding is less.	It binds more tightly to plasma proteins.
Action is fast.	Action is slow and sustained.
Less in colloid (7%).	More in colloid (35%).

MUST KNOW

Reverse T_3 (RT_3)

- Deiodinase D_3 is the main source of RT_3.
- RT_3 is usually elevated in a condition called **"Euthyroid sick syndrome". This condition is associated with** prolonged starvation.

Thyroid Stimulating Hormone

- Thyroid stimulating hormone (TSH) is a glycoprotein hormone.
- Actions of TSH on thyroid gland are as follows:
  - Increases the secretion of thyroid hormones
  - Increases iodide trapping
  - Secretion of thyroglobulin into the colloid
  - Endocytosis of colloid
  - Increases the vascularity of the thyroid gland

Actions of Thyroid Hormones

Thyroid hormones produce all its effects by acting through **nuclear receptor.**

- **Effects on the metabolic rate:**
  - Thyroid hormones increase the basal rate of oxygen consumption (basal metabolic rate) in virtually all the body regions.
  - Thyroid hormones increase the activity of Na K ATPase pump.
  - Because of increase in metabolism, there is increase in heat production by thyroid hormones (thermogenesis).
  - Thyroid hormones stimulate the synthesis of uncoupling proteins (UCP-1) in brown adipose tissue. These proteins dissipate mitochondrial energy gradient as heat rather than ATP formation.
  - Hyperthyroidism is characterized by heat intolerance, whereas hypothyroidism is characterized by cold intolerance.
- **Effects on metabolism**
  - Thyroid hormones are amplifiers of cellular metabolic activity (catabolic).
  - Carbohydrate metabolism: Increases blood glucose
  - Lipid metabolism: Promote lipolysis
  - Protein metabolism: Proteolysis
  - Cholesterol metabolism: Lowers blood cholesterol levels
  - Glycosaminoglycans: Substances like hyaluronic acid and chondroitin sulfate combine with a variety of proteins in skin. Thyroid hormones favor catabolism of such proteins. In hypothyroidism, these complexes hold water and accumulates which is seen as puffiness of skin termed **myxedema.**
- **Effects on the nervous system**
  - Thyroid hormones are very important for normal development of central nervous system.
  - It helps in myelination.
  - Congenital hypothyroidism: One of the most important causes of preventable mental retardation.
- **Effect on bone:** Promote normal growth and skeletal development.
- **Effects on cardiovascular system**
  - Much of the effect of thyroid hormones in heart is due to: Enhancing the responsiveness of heart to circulating catecholamines.

- Increases cardiac output.
- Resting heart rate and the stroke volume are increased (positive chronotropic effect).
- Enhances myocardial contractility (positive inotropic effect).
- Causes cutaneous vasodilation leading to decrease in total peripheral vascular resistance.

- **Effect on respiratory system:** Since the metabolic rate is increased, there is increase in the resting respiratory rate.
- **Effects on gastrointestinal tract**
    - Thyroid hormones increase appetite and food intake. It increases GI motility.
    - Hyperthyroidism is characterized by increase in frequency of bowel movements termed **hyperdefecation** leading to diarrhea.
    - Hypothyroidism is characterized by constipation.
- **Effects on reproductive system**
    - Thyroid hormones are essential for normal sexual function in men and women. They play a permissive role in the regulation of sexual functions.
    - **Hyperthyroidism:** Oligomenorrhea.
    - **Hypothyroidism:** Menorrhagia, loss of libido, infertility.

ENDOCRINE PANCREAS

- The endocrine part of the pancreas comprises a collection of cells termed **islets of Langerhans.** Islets are more plentiful in the tail region of pancreas.

MUST KNOW

Important cells present in endocrine pancreas are as follows:

- A cells (or) Alpha cells—Glucagon
- B cells (or) Beta cells (60–75%)—maximum: Produce Insulin, Amylin, C peptide
- **Pramlintide** is the amylin analog drug useful in the treatment of diabetes mellitus.
- C-peptide is secreted in equimolar amounts to insulin. It is a useful marker of insulin secretion.
- D cells (or) Delta cells: Somatostatin
- F cells: Pancreatic polypeptide

- Cells in islets regulate the secretion of nearby cells (paracrine effect): Glucagon stimulates insulin and somatostatin secretion. Insulin inhibits glucagon secretion. Somatostatin inhibits insulin, glucagon and pancreatic polypeptide.

Glucagon

- Glucagon is a "hyperglycemic hormone". It increases blood glucose and is useful in emergency management of hypoglycemia.
- Glucagon in high concentration increases myocardial contractility without increase in excitability—positive inotropic action: antidote for beta adrenergic blocker overdose.
- Glucagon relaxes intestine. This action of glucagon is used extensively in radiology as an aid to X-ray visualization of bowel.
- **Stimulators of glucagon secretion: Hypoglycemia (most potent),** protein rich meal, alanine, serine, exercise, β-adrenergic stimulation, starvation, stress.
- **Inhibitors of glucagon secretion: Glucose, insulin, somatostatin.**
- **Glucagonoma:** Pancreatic neuroendocrine tumor (pNET), characterized by migratory necrolytic erythema, glucose intolerance/diabetes and weight loss.
- **Mahvash disease:** Due to mutation in human glucagon receptor. **Characterized by** α-cell hyperplasia, hyperglucagonemia.

Insulin

- Nobel Prize in physiology or medicine for discovery of insulin was awarded to **Banting** and **Macleod.**
- It is a polypeptide containing 51 amino acids that are arranged in two chains namely A chain (having 21 amino acids) and B chain (having 30 amino acids).
- Insulin was the first protein whose structure was completely sequenced.
- Human insulin was the first protein to be produced commercially by recombinant DNA technology.
- Transcriptions factors that are essential during synthesis of insulin: Hepatocyte nuclear factor (HNF). Mutation in HNF—**Maturity-onset diabetes of the young** (MODY).
- Zinc stabilizes the structure of insulin. Insulin exists as a hexamer associated with two zinc molecules.
- **The most important stimulus for secretion of insulin is glucose. Glucose acts directly on pancreatic B cells to increase insulin secretion.**

Step 1: Glucose entry: glucose transporter-2 (GLUT-2).
Mutations in glucose transporter GLUT-2 cause
Fanconi Bickel syndrome—characterized by Hyperglycemia

Step 2: Closure of ATP sensitive potassium channel: reduced potassium efflux- Depolarization

Step 3: Opening of voltage gated calcium channel: Entry of calcium ions

Step 4: Exocytosis of insulin, Amylin, C peptide

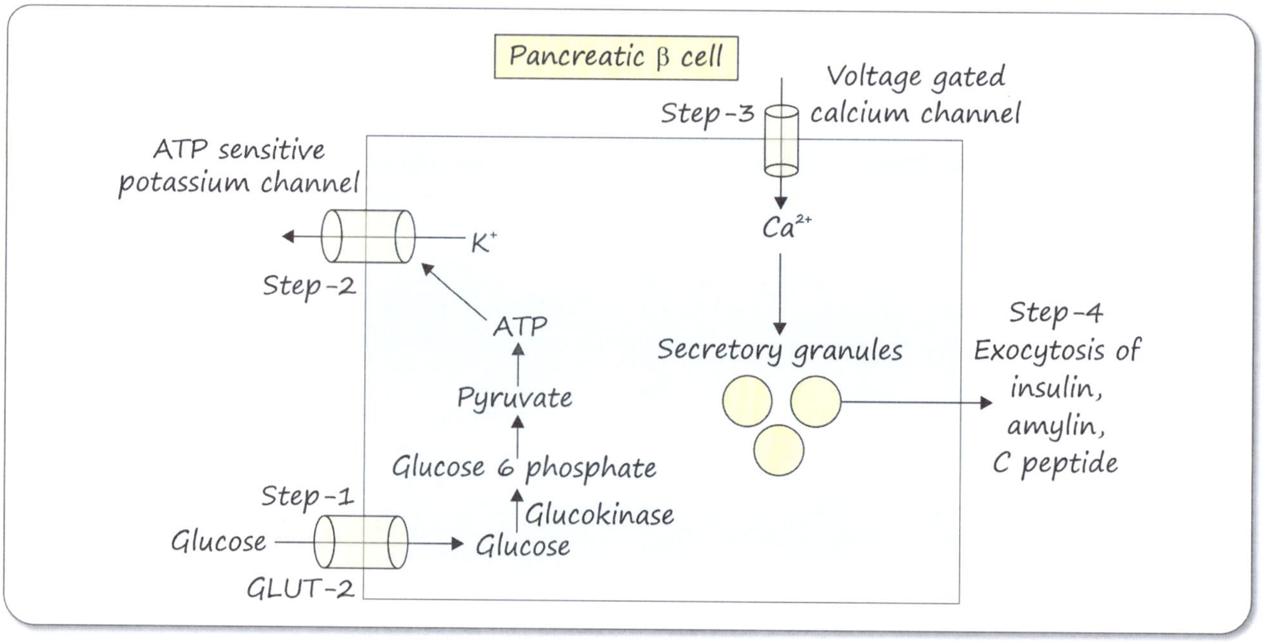

Release of insulin

- Oral hypoglycemic drugs, namely sulfonylurea close ATP sensitive potassium channel leading to insulin secretion.
- **ATP sensitive potassium openers:** Diazoxide-decrease in insulin secretion: the **drug of choice** for pancreatic beta cell tumor **insulinoma.**
- Mutations in ATP sensitive potassium channel cause **persistent hyperinsulinemic hypoglycemia of infancy. Also called "Nesidioblastosis".**

Actions of Insulin

- Insulin acts through tyrosine kinase receptor. The receptor has two alpha subunits and two beta subunits.
- Insulin plays an important role in storage of carbohydrates, lipids and proteins. It is for this action insulin is also called "hormone of abundance": Major ANABOLIC hormone.
- Major actions of insulin are glycogenic, antigluconeogenetic, antilipolytic and nonketotic.
- Insulin increases uptake of glucose into target cells, thereby directing the insertion of glucose transporters **(GLUT 4)** into the cell membranes: This action decreases blood glucose. GLUT 4 is an example of facilitated diffusion.
- Insulin sensitive cells for glucose uptake are skeletal muscle, heart and adipose tissue.
- Insulin causes potassium ions to enter into the cell. This action decreases extracellular potassium levels.
- Pathways stimulated by Insulin: Glycogenesis, lipogenesis, glycolysis.
- Pathways inhibited by Insulin: Glycogenolysis, neoglucogenesis, lipolysis, ketogenesis.
- Insulin inhibits the activity of hormone sensitive lipase and inhibits lipolysis.

Factors that increase insulin secretion	Factors that inhibit insulin secretion

• Glucose—most potent factor
• Glucagon
• Amino acids
  ▪ Arginine and leucine increase insulin secretion
	• Somatostatin
	• Sympathetic discharge
	  ▪ α-Adrenergic stimulators like norepinephrine and epinephrine inhibit insulin secretion

Contd...

Factors that increase insulin secretion	Factors that inhibit insulin secretion
• Long chain fatty acids • Sympathetic discharge ▪ β-Adrenergic stimulators increase insulin secretion • Parasympathetic ▪ Vagal stimulation and acetylcholine increase insulin secretion • Incretin hormones ▪ GI hormones like glucagon-like peptide-1 (GLP-1) and gastric inhibitory peptide (GIP) increase insulin secretion • Theophylline	• β-Adrenergic blockers • Potassium (K^+) depletion • Diazoxide • Thiazide diuretics • Phenytoin • Streptozocin and alloxan ▪ These two are the most prominent diabetogenic chemicals useful in diabetes research (Experimental diabetes)

- Glucagon-like peptide-1 (GLP-1)—most potent incretin.
- Glucagon-like peptide-1 (GLP-1) analogs like Exenatide: useful in treatment of diabetes mellitus
- GLP-1 is rapidly degraded by an enzyme dipeptidyl peptidase-4 (DPP-4). Blockers of DPP-4 prolong the action of GLP-1 and increase insulin.
- DPP-4 blocker useful in the treatment of diabetes mellitus is Sitagliptin.

Hyperglycemic Hormones

Certain hormones antagonize the action of insulin. They produce hyperglycemia. They are also called counter regulatory hormones. Such hyperglycemic hormones are cortisol, growth hormone, glucagon, epinephrine, thyroid hormones.

ADRENAL GLAND

- Adrenal gland is also called suprarenal gland. It consists of two parts namely Adrenal cortex **(72% of gland)** and Adrenal medulla **(28% of gland).**
- Layers of Adrenal cortex
  - Zona glomerulosa (15%): Mineralocorticoids – Aldosterone
  - Zona fasciculata (50%): Glucocorticoids—Cortisol
  - Zona reticularis (7%): Adrenal androgens—Dehydroepiandrosterone
- Adrenal cortical hormones are steroid hormones. They are all derivatives of cholesterol.
- Secretion of cortisol and adrenal sex steroids is completely under the control of Adrenocorticotropic hormone (ACTH) from anterior pituitary. **Corticotropin releasing hormone (CRH)** releases ACTH from anterior pituitary.
- Adrenal medulla: Hormones produced are the catecholamines namely Epinephrine (90%), Norepinephrine (10%), and Dopamine.

ALDOSTERONE

- **Major actions of aldosterone are:**
  - Sodium reabsorption—from urine, sweat, saliva and colon.
  - Water reabsorption (secondary effect)
  - Secretion of potassium ion (K^+)
  - Secretion of H^+ ion in urine (Urinary acidity)
- In the absence of aldosterone, its receptors are kept in inactive state at cytoplasm by binding with chaperone proteins (heat-shock proteins). Once the hormone binds, it gets activated and enters the nucleus. Aldosterone receptor blocker drugs are **spironolactone and eplerenone.**
- Half-life of aldosterone is short. It is about 20 minutes.
- Aldosterone increases sodium reabsorption by increasing the activity of epithelial sodium channels (ENaCs) in principal cells (P cells).
- ENaC blocker drug: Amiloride—useful as diuretic
- **Gain of function mutation of Epithelial sodium channels (ENaCs) – "Liddle syndrome":** Classically manifest severe hypertension with hypokalemia. Treatment: Amiloride
- Aldosterone increases the secretion of potassium ion from principal cell through renal outer medullary potassium (ROMK) channels.
- Aldosterone increases secretion of H^+ ion in urine by stimulating H^+ ATPase present in the membrane of intercalated cells in kidney.

Excessive Production of Aldosterone—"Hyperaldosteronism"

- **Conn's syndrome**
  - Most common cause is aldosterone-producing adrenal adenomas.
  - Excess aldosterone: Sodium and water retention leading to expansion of ECF volume and hypertension.
  - Excess potassium excretion by kidney (K^+ loss).
  - Excessive urinary excretion of H^+ ion leading to metabolic alkalosis.
  - Aldosterone escape phenomenon: In spite of action of aldosterone on the renal tubules, Sodium excretion is increased during aldosterone excess. This is because of the increase in atrial natriuretic peptide (ANP) secretion that excretes sodium in response to increase in ECF volume.

Adrenal Insufficiency (Hypoadrenalism)—"Addison's Disease"

- Due to mineralocorticoid deficiency
  - Hyponatremia (80% of patients)
  - Hyperkalemia
  - Postural hypotension
  - Small heart
- **Hyperpigmentation:** Since ACTH is derived from Pro-opiomelanocortin (POMC), it has some intrinsic melanocyte-stimulating hormone (MSH) action. Very high levels of ACTH in Addison's disease cause hyperpigmentation.

GLUCOCORTICOIDS—"CORTISOL"

- Cortisol is a "stress hormone". It is a lifesaving hormone during stress.
- After release into the circulation, cortisol binds with its binding protein called **corticosteroid-binding globulin (CBG) or transcortin.**
- Half-life of cortisol in the circulation is about **60–90 minutes.**
- In the absence of cortisol, its receptors are kept in inactive state at cytoplasm by binding with chaperone proteins (heat-shock proteins). Once the hormone binds, it gets activated and enters the nucleus.
- Cortisol excess: Cushing syndrome

Actions of cortisol		
Effect	**Mechanism**	**Clinical features in Cushing syndrome (Cortisol excess)**
On carbohydrate metabolism	Cortisol is a "Hyperglycemic hormone". It increases blood glucose mainly by neoglucogenesis.	Glucose intolerance, Diabetes mellitus
On protein metabolism	Cortisol is catabolic to proteins present in the muscle. Cortisol is anabolic in liver. It increases the synthesis of plasma proteins from liver.	Muscle weakness
On fat metabolism	Cortisol is lipolytic.	Dyslipidemia
On immune system	Cortisol is a universal anti-inflammatory agent.	Increased susceptibility to infections
On blood cells	Cortisol decreases the blood levels of eosinophils, lymphocytes, basophils. Cortisol increases the blood levels of neutrophils, monocytes, platelets, RBCs.	Eosinopenia
On nervous system	Cortisol alters mood and behavior. It increases appetite.	Psychosis in severe cases
On heart	Cortisol increases cardiac output. It Increases peripheral vascular tone.	Hypertension
On kidney	It Increase glomerular filtration rate. It increases the excretion of calcium.	Hypercalciuria
On bone	Cortisol increases bone resorption by increasing activity of osteoclasts	Osteoporosis (vertebral fractures)

Contd...

Effect	Mechanism	Clinical features in Cushing syndrome (Cortisol excess)
On connective tissues	Cortisol inhibits fibroblast proliferation and collagen formation	Easy bruising, Delayed wound healing, purple stretch marks
On GI tract	Cortisol increases gastric acid secretion.	Peptic ulcers
On reproductive system	It inhibits the secretion of GnRH.	In women—amenorrhea, infertility. In men—loss of libido, impotence.

ADRENAL SEX STEROIDS

- Adrenal sex steroids produced from zona reticularis are Dehydroepiandrosterone (DHEA)—major one, Dehydroepiandrosterone sulfate (DHEAS), Androstenedione and Testosterone—only small amounts
- Since males have more active androgens testosterone and dihydrotestosterone, adrenal androgens have only weak effects.
- In **females**, active androgens contribute about 50% of circulating active androgens and are required for axillary hair growth, pubic hair growth, libido.
- **Adrenogenital Syndrome**
  - Usually occurs due to an adrenocortical tumor that secretes excessive adrenal androgens.
  - The predominant feature due to excessive adrenal androgens is **Virilization.**
  - In females, **it causes female pseudo-hermaphroditism**. Its clinical features are growth of beard, deeper voice, hirsutism, clitoromegaly.
  - In prepubertal boys, there is rapid development of male sexual **organs (precocious pseudopuberty).**

CALCIUM HOMEOSTASIS

- Normal serum calcium levels are 8.7–10.2 mg/dL.
- Free calcium or ionized calcium: Around 50% of total calcium- responsible for all the important actions of calcium.
- Protein bound calcium: Remaining 50% of total calcium-inactive form.
- **pH changes and calcium levels**
  - Alkalosis (increase in pH) increases the protein bound calcium. This can lead to hypocalcemic tetany (decrease in free calcium).
  - Acidosis (decrease in pH) decreases protein bound calcium and increases the free calcium leading to hypercalcemia.
- **Factors affecting absorption of calcium from GI tract**
  - Absorption of calcium is facilitated by gastric acid and proteins in diet.
  - Absorption of calcium is inhibited by phytates, phosphates, oxalates, fatty acids in diet.
- Three major hormones that regulate calcium levels are parathormone, vitamin D and calcitonin.
- Three major body organs that aid in regulation of calcium levels are bone, intestine and kidney.

PARATHORMONE

- Parathormone (PTH) is a large protein hormone containing 84 amino acids.
- Chief cells synthesize and secrete PTH.
- Calcium acting through **Calcium sensing receptor (CaSR)** inhibits PTH secretion.
- Cinacalcet is the calcimimetic drug that activates the calcium-sensing receptor (CaSR). This action ultimately inhibits PTH secretion.
- Familial hypocalciuric hypercalcemia (FHH) is due to inactivating mutations of CaSR.

Actions of Parathormone

- **In bone**
  - Parathormone (PTH) receptors are only present in osteoblasts.
  - PTH activates osteoblasts which secrete RANKL that aids in differentiation of osteoclasts.
  - Osteoclast mediated bone resorption ultimately increases serum calcium levels.
  - Intermittent administration of PTH leads to a net stimulation of bone formation rather than bone breakdown.

- Intermittent administration of PTH is used to prevent bone resorption in osteoporosis. The drug is called "**Teriparatide**". **This drug is** recombinant form of PTH 1-34.

- **In kidney**
  - Increase calcium resorption from distal tubules through TRPV5
  - PTH increases phosphate excretion by inhibiting the sodium-phosphate cotransporter (NaPi-IIa) in proximal convoluted tubule: "**phosphaturic action**"
- **In intestine**
  - In intestine, action of PTH is indirect.
  - PTH increases calcium absorption in the intestine by stimulating the production of Vitamin D.

Overall action of parathormone is increase in calcium and decrease in phosphate.

VITAMIN D

- The active form of vitamin D is called 1,25-dihydroxycholecalciferol or calcitriol.
- Vitamin D synthesis occurs by the action of ultraviolet (UV) rays on skin. The precursor present in skin on which UV-B rays act is called 7-dehydrocholesterol.
- 7-dehydrocholesterol is converted to Vitamin D_3 or cholecalciferol by the action of UV-B rays.
- In the liver, Vitamin D_3 is 25-hydroxylated by an enzyme called 25-Hydroxylase. The product from liver is called 25-hydroxycholecalciferol or calcidiol. This product is useful to assess vitamin D status in human body.
- 25-hydroxycholecalciferol is converted in the cells of the proximal tubules of the kidneys to the active product called **1,25-dihydroxycholecalciferol or calcitriol.**
- The enzyme responsible for this hydroxylation is called **1α-Hydroxylase.** Rate limiting step in vitamin D synthesis is the formation of calcitriol by the enzyme 1α-Hydroxylase.
- Major inducers of 1α-Hydroxylase enzyme are PTH and hypophosphatemia.
- Major inhibitors of 1α-Hydroxylase enzyme are calcium, FGF23 and the product calcitriol itself (negative feedback).

Actions of Vitamin D

- **In intestine**
  - Increases intestinal absorption of calcium by increasing calbindin (calcium-binding protein).
  - Increases calcium transporters namely TRPV5 and TRPV6 (transient receptor potential vanilloid).
- **In bone**
  - **D = Dual.** Causes both bone formation and bone resorption depending on serum calcium levels.
  - Vitamin D receptor is present in osteoblasts.
  - Vitamin D activates osteoblasts which secretes RANKL that aids in differentiation of osteoclasts. Osteoclast mediated bone resorption ultimately increases serum calcium levels.
- **In Kidney**
  - It facilitates Ca^{2+} reabsorption in the kidneys by increasing TRPV5 expression in the distal tubules.
  - It also increases phosphate reabsorption from proximal tubules.
- Overall action of Vitamin D is increase in calcium and phosphate.

CALCITONIN

- Calcium lowering hormone produced from the parafollicular C cells of the thyroid gland.
- Calcitonin receptors are present in osteoclasts.
- It inhibits bone resorption by inhibiting osteoclasts and decreases serum calcium.
- In kidney—it increases the excretion of calcium in urine.
- During pregnancy and lactation—calcitonin prevents excess calcium loss.
- Salcatonin: calcitonin drug useful in treatment of Paget's disease.
- Calcitonin serves as tumor marker for medullary carcinoma of thyroid.

Parathyroid hormone-related protein (PTHrP): PTHrP is responsible for hypercalcemia of malignancy seen in squamous cell carcinoma of the lung.

MUST KNOW

Bone formation (Osteoblast derived) markers are,

1. Amino terminal propeptide of type I collagen (PINP)—most preferred
2. Carboxy terminal propeptide of type I collagen (PICP)
3. Osteocalcin
4. Bone specific alkaline phosphatase

MUST KNOW

Bone resorption (Osteoclast derived) markers are,

1. C-telopeptide (CTX)
2. N-telopeptide (NTX)
3. Pyridinoline (PYO)
4. Deoxypyridinoline (DVD)

REPRODUCTIVE PHYSIOLOGY

Sex-determining Region of the Y Chromosome (SRY)

- Located near the tip of the short arm of Y chromosome.
- Also called testis-determining gene product. Presence of SRY alone is sufficient for the gonad to develop into testis.
- SRY increases the production of two hormones from testis. They are testosterone—from Leydig cells—and Anti-Müllerian hormone (AMH) also called Müllerian inhibiting substance (MIS)—from Sertoli cells.

Puberty

- Most important event associated with puberty is increase in pulsatile release of gonadotropin hormone releasing hormone (GnRH). Puberty is characterized by nocturnal luteinizing hormone (LH) pulses in children.
- Before puberty, the pulsatile release of GnRH is inhibited by GABA, Melatonin.
- Exactly around the time of puberty, pulsatile release of GnRH is initiated by kisspeptin.
- Kisspeptin, also called **metastin,** acts through its G protein–coupled receptor called GPR54 present in GnRH neurons.
- Children with mutations in GPR54 fail to enter puberty.
- The timing of the onset of puberty is usually correlated with adequate body fat reserves.
- Permissive role of leptin: Hormone produced by adipose cells, termed leptin, signals the adequate body stores to brain and aids the GnRH pulsatile release.

Male Reproduction

Spermatogenesis

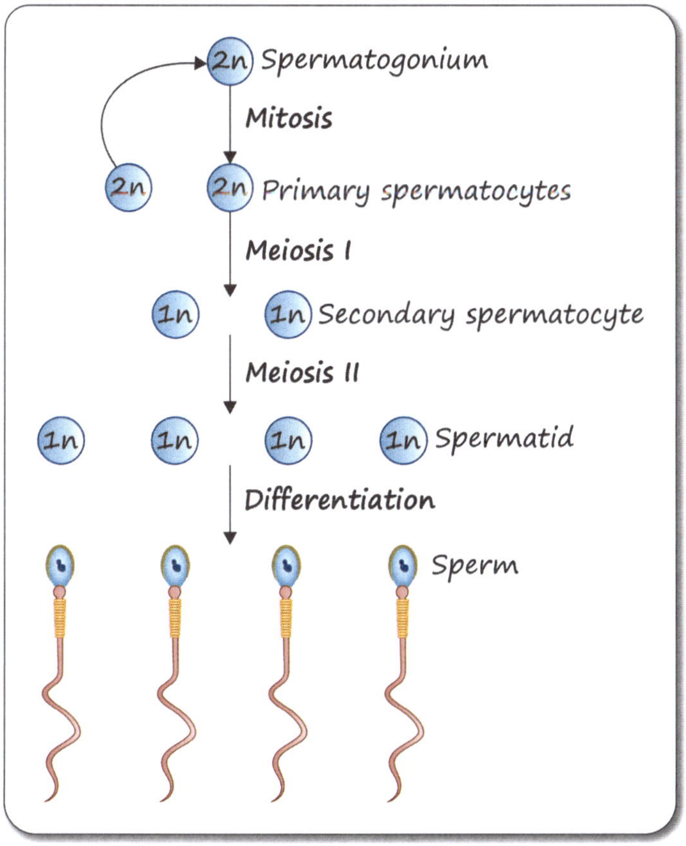

- The process of spermatogenesis takes about 74 days
- Spermatogonia undergoes mitotic divisions to form primary spermatocytes
- Primary spermatocytes undergo first meiotic division to form secondary spermatocytes
- Secondary spermatocytes undergo second meiotic division to form four spermatids
- Spermatids become mature spermatozoza: **"Spermiogenesis"**
- **Spermiation** is the process where sperm is released
- Velocity of human sperm movement is 1–4 mm/min
- The life span of ejaculated sperm in the female genital tract is only 1 to 2 days
- Maturation of sperm takes place in epididymis
- Forward progressive motility of sperm requires activation of a Ca^{2+} channel called **CatSper**
- Capacitation of sperm: Occurs mainly in the female genital tract (uterus)
- During capacitation, forward motility of sperm increases, facilitation of acrosome reaction occurs

Leydig Cells

- Leydig cells are the steroidogenic stromal cells that synthesize and secrete testosterone.
- Luteinizing hormone (LH) acts in Leydig cells to increase the secretion of testosterone.

Sertoli Cells

- During development, Sertoli cells produce anti-Mullerian hormone (AMH) that induces the regression of Mullerian duct in male.
- Adjacent Sertoli cells form blood-testis barrier, which is an immunologically safe microenvironment for developing sperm.
- Provides nutrients to the developing spermatozoa. Sertoli cells are also called "Nurse cells of testis".
- Sertoli cells produce androgen-binding protein (ABP) that binds testosterone.
- It has the enzyme aromatase that converts testosterone to estrogen.
- Sertoli cells produce the hormone inhibin which inhibits pituitary FSH.
- Sertoli cells perform phagocytic function—they engulf dead sperm cells.
- Sertoli cell functions are regulated by FSH—through FSH receptor.

Semen

- Semen is comprised of secretions from Seminal vesicle—almost 60 percent of volume, Prostate—20 to 30% and Vas deferens — 10%.
- Seminal vesicle secretions contain fructose, ascorbic acid, prostaglandins and phosphoryl-choline.
- Prostate secretions contain spermine, fibrinolysin and acid phosphatase.
- Important buffers present in semen are phosphate and bicarbonate.
- **Tests to identify seminal stains**
  - **Florence test:** Choline is detected in this method.
  - **Barberio test:** Spermine is detected in this method.

Male Sexual Act

- Involves erection of penis, ejaculation and finally detumescence.
- **Erection of penis**
  - Mediated by Parasympathetic nerve fibers from S2–S4 sacral spinal segments, Nitric oxide mediated vascular relaxation and Prostaglandin mediated vascular relaxation.
  - Involves increased flow of blood, compression of veins and accumulation of blood in the corpora cavernosa.
  - **Treatment of erectile dysfunction:** Phosphodiesterase type 5 (PDE-5) inhibitors like sildenafil, Prostaglandin analogs like Alprostadil.
- **Ejaculation**
  - Stimulated by the sympathetic nervous system.
  - Involves emission of semen into urethra which is followed by rhythmic contractions of the bulbocavernosus and ischiocavernosus muscles, leading to ejaculation.
  - **Retrograde ejaculation:** When the internal urethral sphincter does not close. Seen in men with diabetes.
- **Detumescence:** Penis returns to the flaccid state. Mediated by norepinephrine and endothelin.

Regulation of Male Reproductive Functions

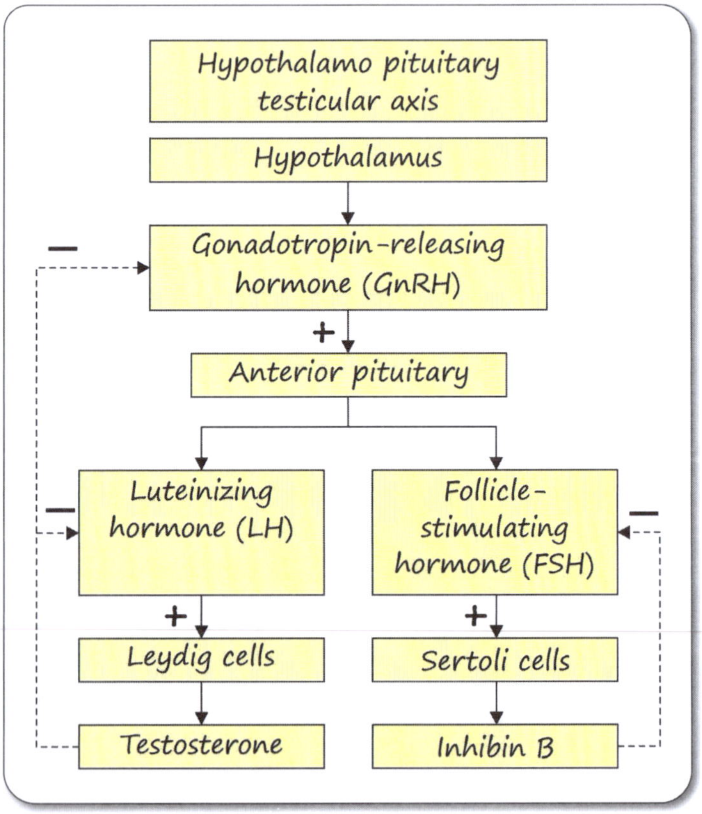

Testosterone

- Principal androgen hormone of the testes produced by Leydig cells.
- Testosterone is a C_{19} steroid.

- In circulation, testosterone binds with Gonadal steroid-binding globulin (GBG) or Sex Hormone-binding globulin (SHBG)—65% and Albumin—33%.
- The remaining 2% is free testosterone—it is the biologically active form.
- Actions are mediated through androgen receptor (AR).
- During development, testosterone plays an important role in stimulation of **Wolffian duct** leading to the formation of **male internal genitalia.**
- Stimulates erythropoietin synthesis: Increase in RBC count in men.
- Initiation and maintenance of spermatogenesis.
- Stimulates bone growth.
- Has protein anabolic effects—increases the rate of growth and increase in muscle mass.

Dihydrotestosterone (DHT)

- Formed from testosterone by the action of an enzyme 5α-reductase.
- DHT is mainly responsible for many of the changes associated with puberty in boys.
- DHT is very important for masculinization of the **external genitalia** and development of the **prostate gland.**
- It is responsible for facial hair, acne and the temporal recession of the hairline in males.
- Finasteride and Dutasteride are 5α-reductase inhibitors. These drugs are mainly useful in treatment of **benign prostatic hyperplasia** (BPH).

Female Reproduction

Oogenesis

- Refers to the process of formation of ova from the primitive germ cells.
- In humans, no new ova are formed after birth.

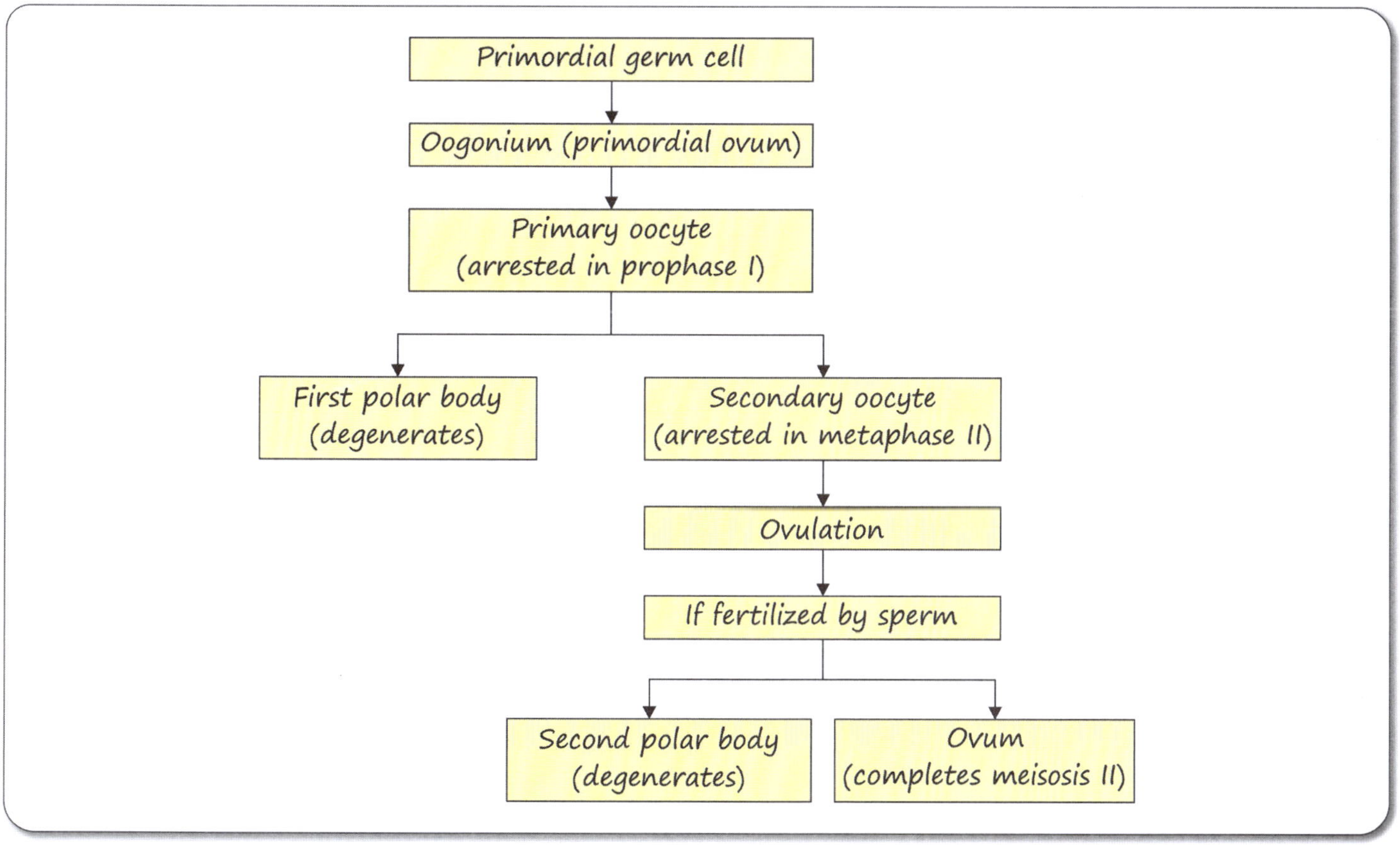

The Menstrual Cycle

- Menstrual cycle refers to the regular cyclical changes that occur every month. Duration is 28 days.
- Such cyclical changes are seen in the form of ovarian cycle, uterine endometrial cycle, uterine cervix cycle and vaginal cycle.

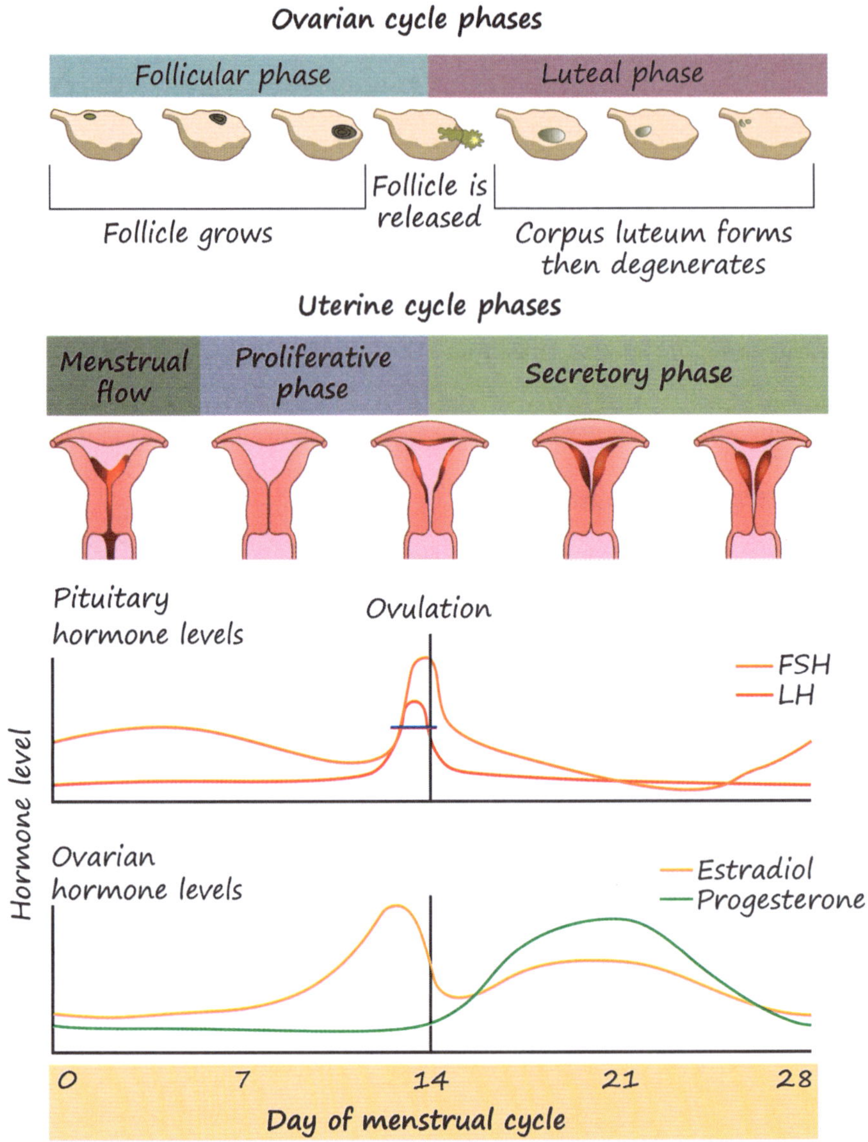

Ovarian Cycle

Consists of the following phases: pre-ovulatory phase or follicular phase, ovulation and post-ovulatory phase or luteal phase.

1. Follicular Phase

- Starts from the fifth day of the cycle till the time of ovulation (usually happens at 14th day of the cycle).
- 15–20 follicles are selected and they mature under the influence of Follicle Stimulating Hormone (FSH).
- Dominant follicle: It is the largest follicle characterized by maximum FSH receptors, highest antral concentration of estrogen and Inhibin A and high aromatase activity.

2. Ovulation

- Process of release of ovum that happens around 14th day of the cycle.
- A surge of Luteinizing Hormone (LH) is necessary for ovulation: Exactly around 24-36 hours before ovulation, estrogen increases the levels of LH. This is an example of positive feedback.
- LH reaches its peak value around 8-12 hours before ovulation, termed **LH peak.**
- There is also a rise in FSH (FSH surge) around the time of ovulation. This rise in FSH is responsible for increase in plasmin that helps in lysis of wall of the follicle.

3. Luteal Phase

- Constant period of about 14 days.

- Characterized by formation of **Corpus haemorrhagicum:** Outer wall of the Graafian follicle collapses and fills with blood.
- **Corpus luteum:** The clotted blood is rapidly replaced with yellowish lipid-rich luteal cells.
- Luteinizing hormone is responsible for luteinization: causes rapid secretion of the steroid hormone **progesterone.**
- If there is no fertilization of ovum—corpus luteum regresses by about 24th day of cycle and is replaced by a whitish scar tissue—corpus albicans.
- If there is fertilization of ovum—corpus luteum is maintained and it serves as the major source for estrogen and progesterone till 3rd month of pregnancy.

Uterine Endometrial Cycle

Divided into three phases namely Proliferative phase—6th to 14th day then Secretory phase—15th to 28th day and finally Menstrual phase—1st to 5th day.

1. Proliferative Phase

- Proliferative phase is about **restoration of the lost epithelium.**
- Endometrium increases rapidly in thickness under the influence of estrogen.
- Uterine glands lengthen but they do not secrete.

2. Secretory Phase

- Secretory phase is about **preparation for implantation.**
- Starts after ovulation.
- The thickness of the endometrium reaches its highest (6–8 mm).
- The uterine glands become coiled and tortuous and they begin to secrete a clear fluid. The blood vessels undergo marked spiraling.

3. Menstrual Phase

- Superficial two-thirds of the endometrium (stratum functionale) is shed during menstruation.
- Major reason for menstrual bleed is the regression of corpus luteum (hormonal support is lost). This leads to spasm and degeneration of the spiral arteries that causes menstrual flow. Such vasospasm is usually caused by prostaglandin $F_{2\alpha}$ ($PGF_{2\alpha}$).

Cyclical Changes in Uterine Cervix

- Estrogen makes the cervical mucus thinner and more alkaline—promote the survival and transport of sperm.
- Fern pattern: due to **high sodium chloride** and low protein content in the mucus due to **high estrogen.**
- **Spinnbarkeit:** Increased elasticity of cervical mucus due to high estrogen level and the mucus is stretchable.
- Progesterone—makes cervical mucus thick and tenacious.
- Cervical mucus is thinnest at the time of ovulation.

Cyclical Changes in Vagina

- The exfoliated vaginal epithelial cells normally include:
  - Parabasal cells—lack of hormonal activity
  - Intermediate cells—predominates under progesterone influence
  - Superficial cells—predominates under estrogen influence

Regulation of Female Reproductive Functions

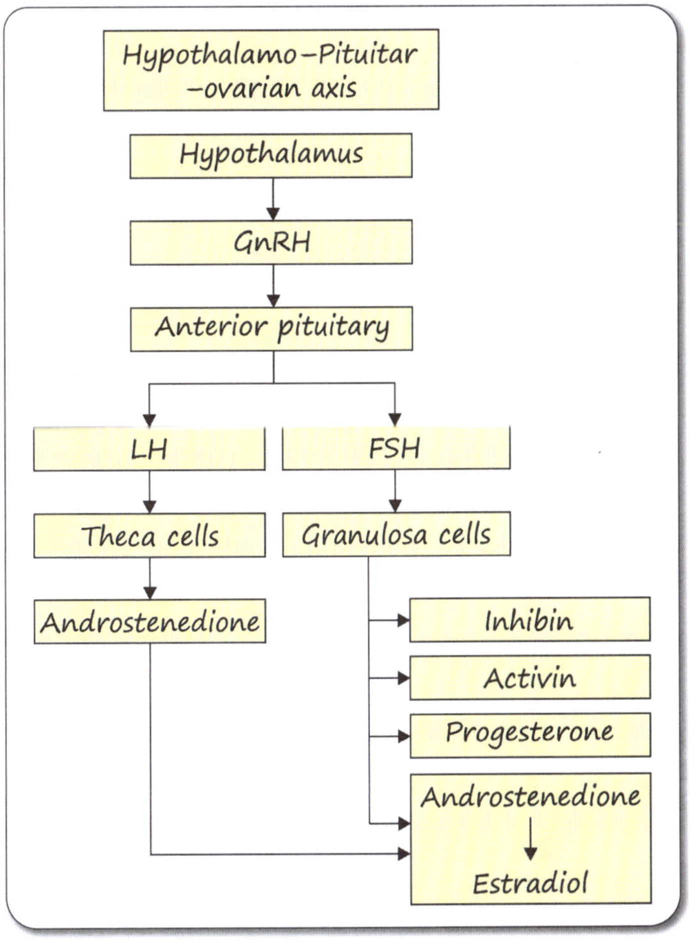

MUST KNOW

Two Cell – Two Gonadotropin Model

- Two cells: Theca cells and Granulosa cells.
- Two Gonadotropins: Luteinizing hormone (LH) and Follicle Stimulating Hormone (FSH).
- LH acts on theca cells to increase the production of androstenedione.
- Granulosa cells convert this androstenedione to estradiol with the help of an enzyme "aromatase".
- Estradiol and progesterone always inhibit LH (negative feedback).
- Inhibin inhibits FSH secretion.

Female Reproductive Hormones

- Steroid hormones: Estrogen, Progesterone
- Protein/Peptide Hormones: Activin, Inhibin, Relaxin

1. Steroid Hormones

Estrogen

- C18 steroids
- Naturally occurring estrogens are:
    - Estradiol (E2)—predominant estrogen during reproductive years.
    - Estrone (E1)—predominant estrogen in menopausal women.
    - Estriol (E3)—predominant estrogen in pregnant women.
- Major binding proteins for estradiol are Albumin —60% and Gonadal steroid-binding globulin (GBG) or Sex Hormone-binding globulin (SHBG) —38%

Actions of estrogen:

Effects on	Effects of estrogen
Uterus	"Estrogen-dominated" uterus has: • Increased uterine blood flow • Increased content of contractile proteins in uterine smooth muscle • Uterine muscle more active and excitable
Secondary sexual characteristics	• Promotes female body contour • Female distribution of fat in the breasts and buttocks
Breasts	• Promotes mainly ductal growth in breast • "Growth hormone of breast"
Bone	• Promotes survival of osteoblasts • Induces apoptosis of osteoclasts • Inhibits activity of osteoclasts by inhibiting RANKL and increasing the production of **osteoprotegerin** • Loss of estrogen at menopause—leads to osteoporosis
Liver	• "Plasma cholesterol lowering action"
CVS	• Estrogen promotes vasodilation by increasing nitric oxide • inhibits platelet activation
CNS	• Estrogen is "neuroprotective"
Kidney	• Promotes salt and water retention

Progesterone

- C_{21} steroid
- Major sources of progesterone are corpus luteum and placenta.

Actions of progesterone:

Effects on	Effects of progesterone
Uterus	Antiestrogenic effect on the myometrial cells—decreasing in excitability, decrease in sensitivity to oxytocin
Breast	Progesterone stimulates the development of lobules and alveoli
On CNS	Acts as a depressant on the CNS Set-point for thermoregulation is increased—"Thermogenic action" responsible for increase in basal body temperature around ovulation
On kidney	Large doses of progesterone—natriuresis by blocking aldosterone
On respiration	Stimulates respiration. This leads low alveolar PCO_2 during luteal phase of menstrual cycle

2. Peptide Hormones

- **Activin:** Stimulates the synthesis and secretion of FSH.
- **Inhibin:**
  - Inhibits FSH secretion from pituitary cells.
  - Inhibin A is major secretory product of the corpus luteum.
  - Inhibin B is produced mainly by granulosa cells.
- **Follistatin:** Inhibits FSH secretion.
- **Relaxin:** During pregnancy—relaxes the pubic symphysis, softens, and dilates the uterine cervix—facilitates delivery.

PLACENTAL PROTEIN HORMONE: HUMAN CHORIONIC GONADOTROPIN (HCG)

- Mainly produced by syncytiotrophoblast.
- Glycoprotein made up of alpha and beta subunits.
- Alpha subunit similar to LH, FSH and TSH.
- It acts on the same receptor as LH. hCG- 80X the biological activity of LH. hCG = SUPER LH
- Half-life of hCG is about 36 hours.
- Functions of hCG:
  - It rescues and maintains corpus luteum till 6 weeks of pregnancy—major function.
  - Stimulates the secretion of progesterone by the corpus luteum of pregnancy.
  - Stimulates Leydig cells to produce testosterone.
  - Promotes secretion of hormone relaxin from corpus luteum.
  - It is immunosuppressive—inhibits rejection of fetus by the mother.

LACTATION

- Involves four stages namely Mammogenesis, Lactogenesis, Galactokinesis and Galactopoiesis.
  1. **Mammogenesis**
     - Preparation of breast for lactation.
     - Estrogen promotes the growth of ductal system.
     - Progesterone promotes the growth of lobuloalveolar system.
  2. **Lactogenesis**
     - Synthesis and secretion of milk.
     - Hormones involved: Prolactin (most important), Insulin, Growth hormone.
  3. **Galactokinesis**
     - Ejection of milk.
     - Most important hormone responsible for milk ejection is oxytocin.
     - Suckling initiates this reflex. This reflex is called "milk let down reflex". It is an example of a neuroendocrine reflex. This reflex is inhibited by pain and anxiety.
  4. **Galactopoiesis:** Maintenance of lactation—prolactin is solely responsible.

8. RENAL PHYSIOLOGY

STRUCTURE OF KIDNEY AND ITS FUNCTIONS

- The functional unit of kidney is the nephron.
- Each human kidney has approximately 1 million nephrons.
- Kidney essentially performs four important functions, which are glomerular filtration, tubular reabsorption, tubular secretion and excretion.

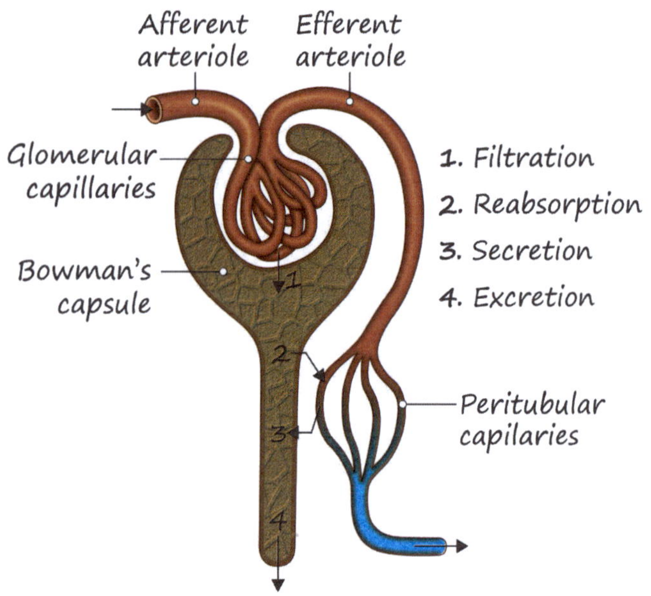

GLOMERULAR FILTRATION RATE

- Normal glomerular filtration rate (GFR) = 125 mL/min or 180 L/day
- Glomerular filtration is called ultrafiltration because the **plasma proteins are not filtered.**
- Proteins are not filtered because of the following reasons:
    - **Charge:** Proteins are anions with negative charge. Polyanionic proteoglycans (heparan sulfate)—repels protein albumin. Positively charged molecules are filtered more readily than negatively charged molecules.
    - **Size:** Glomerular membrane permits neutral substances up to 4 nm in diameter. Substances greater than 8 nm diameter are totally excluded. Glomerular capillaries are fenestrated capillaries.
    - **Slit diaphragm:** Filtration slit is bridged by a thin diaphragm. This slit diaphragm serves as the barrier for filtration of proteins. Important proteins of the slit diaphragm are Nephrin, Podocin and α-actinin 4.
    - Nephrin is coded by NPHS1. Mutation in NPHS1 gene—causes "**congenital nephrotic syndrome of the Finnish type**".
    - Podocin is encoded by NPHS2 gene. Mutation in NPHS2 gene—causes "**steroid-resistant nephrotic syndrome of childhood onset**".
    - Mutations in genes encoding α-actinin 4 cause "**autosomal dominant Focal Segmental Glomerulo Sclerosis (FSGS)**".

Determinants of GFR

- Pressures in the capillaries are the major forces that govern fluid movement in them. Such forces are commonly called Starling forces.
- **Forces Favoring Filtration (mm Hg):** Glomerular hydrostatic pressure = 60
- **Forces Opposing Filtration (mm Hg):** Glomerular capillary colloid osmotic pressure = 32 and Bowman's capsule hydrostatic pressure = 18
- **Net filtration pressure = Forces Favoring Filtration – Forces Opposing Filtration**
- **Net filtration pressure = 60–18–32 = 10 mm Hg**

Measurement of GFR

- "Inulin clearance" is used to estimate GFR because inulin is freely filtered, neither reabsorbed nor secreted by the tubules, biologically inert and non-toxic.
- Inulin clearance test is the gold standard method for estimation of GFR.
- Clearance = U*V/P
- Inulin clearance = 126 mL/min
- Plasma creatinine (P_{Cr}) is the **most widely used marker for GFR.**
- If clearance = GFR means No reabsorption/ secretion. Example is inulin.
- If clearance > GFR means Net secretion. Example is **Para-aminohippuric acid (PAH).**
- If clearance < GFR means Net reabsorption. Example is Glucose.
- Since creatinine is secreted by the tubules, its clearance is slightly higher than inulin.

- **Emerging new markers of GFR:** Cystatin C, β-Trace protein (BTP).

MUST KNOW

Renal Circulation

- Kidneys receive 1.2–1.3 L of blood per minute, or about 23% of the cardiac output.
- **Out of this total renal blood flow, 55% is renal plasma flow (RPF).**
- RPF is 625 mL/min.
- **Estimation of renal plasma flow (RPF) is by "Para-aminohippuric acid (PAH) clearance".**
- Only 90% (0.9) of the plasma PAH is extracted by kidney – the RPF calculated from the clearance of PAH is referred to as the **effective RPF (ERPF).**
- **True (actual) RPF = 625/0.9 = 700 mL/min**

Filtration Fraction

- The filtration fraction (FF) is the ratio of GFR to the renal plasma flow (RPF).
- FF = 125/625 = 0.2 (20%)
- Substances used to measure filtration fraction: for GFR estimation—inulin is used; and for RPF estimation—Para-aminohippuric acid (PAH) is used.

Changes in GFR

Changes in the resistance of afferent and/or efferent arterioles—their effects on Renal Blood Flow (RBF) and GFR are noted.

Arterioles	GFR	RBF
Constriction of afferent arteriole: Example: Norepinephrine, shock	Decreases	Decreases
Constriction of Efferent arteriole—Example: Angiotensin II	Biphasic response. Initially GFR increases, later falls	Decreases
Dilatation of afferent arteriole—Example: Prostaglandins PGE2	Increases	Increases
Dilatation of Efferent arteriole—Example: ACE inhibitors	Decreases	Increases

Regulation of GFR

- The factors that regulate GFR are autoregulation and mesangial cells—by contraction or relaxation.
- Autoregulation mechanisms are Myogenic mechanism and Tubuloglomerular feedback mechanism.

Autoregulation

- Intrinsic ability of an organ to regulate its own blood flow.
- Renal autoregulation is present even in denervated and in isolated, perfused kidneys.
- Mean arterial pressure between 80 mm Hg and 180 mm Hg; renal blood flow and GFR are maintained relatively constant.
- Myogenic mechanism: Increase in blood flow stretches the elastic wall of the afferent arteriole. Stretching leads to increase in calcium influx—vasoconstriction that decreases blood flow.
- Tubuloglomerular Feedback: Macula densa plays an important role. In response to increase in Nacl, macula densa releases the mediator adenosine. Adenosine acts in afferent arteriole to cause vasoconstriction leading to decrease in RBF and GFR.

Mesangial cells—their Role in Regulation of GFR

- **Mesangial cell contraction:** Effect is decrease in GFR.
- **Mesangial cell relaxation:** Effect is increase in GFR.
- **Agents that cause mesangial cell contraction:** Angiotensin-II, Endothelins, Norepinephrine.
- **Agents that cause mesangial cell relaxation:** cAMP, Dopamine, Atrial natriuretic peptide (ANP), Prostaglandins, Nitric oxide.

PARTS OF NEPHRON

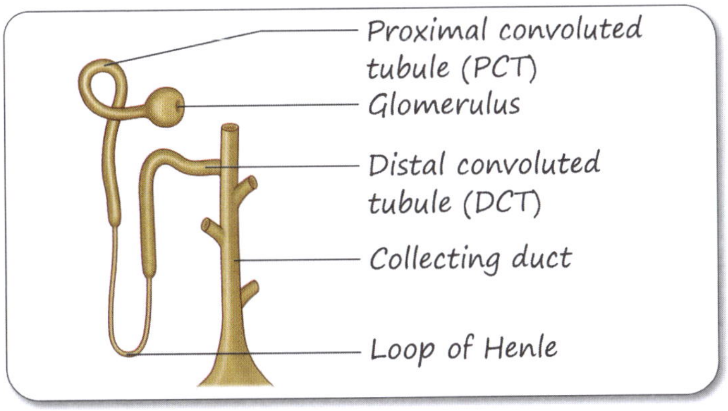

Proximal Convoluted Tubule

- Proximal convoluted tubule (PCT) is the segment of nephron having maximum reabsorption capacity.
- Have brush border on the apical side that increases surface area for reabsorption.
- Have large number of mitochondria—to support active transport processes.
- **Proximal convoluted tubule (PCT) reabsorbs:**
  - 2/3rd (67%) of filtered sodium chloride (NaCl)
  - 2/3rd (67%) of filtered water
  - 2/3rd (67%) of filtered potassium (K^+)
  - 70% of filtered calcium
  - 80% of filtered phosphate and bicarbonate
  - 100% of filtered glucose and amino acids
- 60% of sodium reabsorption is mainly through Na H antiport.
- Another major transport protein for sodium is sodium glucose cotransporter (SGLT-2).
- Other important sodium transporters in PCT are Na^+/Pi cotransporter, Na+ amino acid cotransporter.

Glucose Reabsorption in PCT

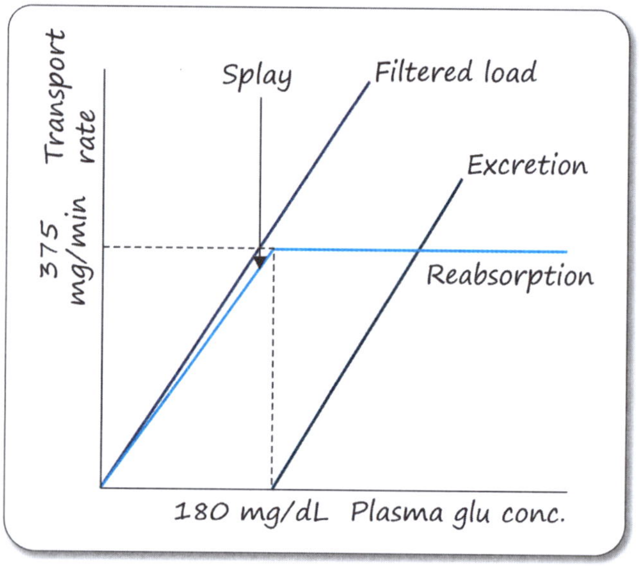

- **PCT reabsorbs 100% of filtered glucose**
- Glucose is resorbed along with sodium in PCT through sodium glucose cotransporter (SGLT-2)
- **Transport maximum of glucose (TmG):** Refers to the point where glucose carrier proteins in PCT are fully saturated
- TmG is 375 mg/min
- **Renal threshold** for glucose: The plasma level at which the glucose first appears in the urine in more than the normal minute amounts
- Renal threshold for glucose is 180 mg/dL
- Splay: deviation noted in reabsorption curve
- The reason for this deviation is that all the nephrons do not have the same filtering and reabsorbing capacities for glucose
- Sodium glucose cotransporter 2 (SGLT-2) blocker drugs are **Canagliflozin, Dapagliflozin**
- They are useful in treatment of diabetes mellitus

Tubular Fluid (TF)/Plasma (P) or TF/P Ratio

- TF/P: To find out the changes in concentrations of various solutes along the proximal tubule.
- If TF/P = 1, then that substance is equally reabsorbed with water. Such TF/P = 1 is seen for sodium and osmolarity.
- If TF/P is >1, then that substance is reabsorbed proportionately less than water. Such TF/P >1 is seen for chloride, inulin, urea and creatinine.
- If TF/P is <1, then that substance is reabsorbed proportionately more than water. Such TF/P <1 is seen for Glucose, amino acids, and HCO_3^-

Loop of Henle

- Loop of Henle reabsorbs 25 % of the filtered load of NaCl, 15% of the filtered load of water, 20% of the filtered load of calcium and 10% of the filtered load of bicarbonate.
- Loop of Henle plays an important role in concentration of urine through **countercurrent mechanism.**
- A countercurrent system is a system of U-shaped tubes in which the flow of fluid is in opposite direction in two limbs of the U-shaped tubules.
- **Countercurrent system locations:** Kidney—loop of Henle, limbs, testis, intestine.

Descending loop of Henle
concentrating segment

- The fluid leaves out of PCT is isosmotic (300 mOsm/kg)
- In descending loop of Henle (dLOH), water moves out freely leaving the solutes inside
- Fluid becomes **hypertonic**
- The osmolarity reached at the tip of dLOH is around 1200 mOsm/kg

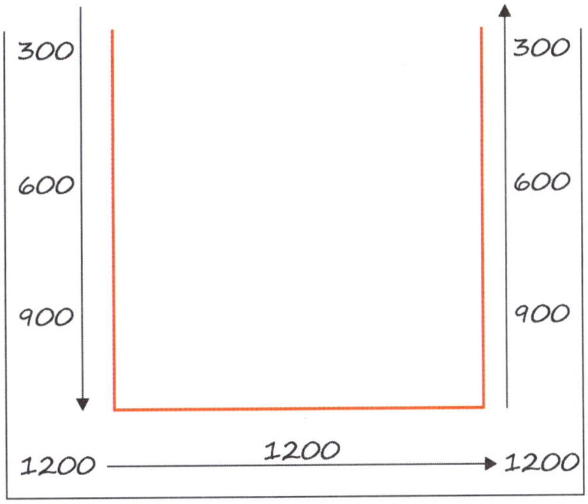

Asending loop of Henle
diluting segment

- Thick ascending loop of Henle is permeable to solutes and impermeable to water
- Sodium, chloride and potassium move out of the thick ascending limb through Na-K-2Cl cotransporter
- Fluid becomes hypotonic

- ***Countercurrent exchanger—"Vasa recta":*** *they minimize washout of solutes and maintain the osmolarity gradient developed by the loop of Henle.*
- ***Recycling of potassium into ascending loop of Henle:*** *Lumen positivity: Helps in reabsorption of calcium, magnesium.*
- *Remember that only 50% of medullary hyperosmolarity is due to NaCl. Remaining 50% is contributed by the end product of protein metabolism—urea*
- *High protein diet increases the concentrating ability of kidney; and low protein diet decreases the ability of kidneys to concentrate the urine.*
- ***Drugs that block Na-K-2Cl cotransporter in thick ascending loop of Henle—"Loop diuretics":*** *Furosemide.*
- *Bartter syndrome: Autosomal recessive (AR) type I: Mutation in Na-K-2Cl cotransporter.*
- *Bartter syndrome: AR type IV: Mutation in subunit of chloride (Barttin).*
- *Clinical features of Bartter syndrome are Hypokalemia, Metabolic alkalosis, Hyper-aldosteronism, Hypercalciuria—renal stones.*

Distal Convoluted Tubule

- ***Major role of distal convoluted tubule (DCT): Reabsorption of*** *5% of filtered load of NaCl, 9% of filtered load of calcium.*
- ***NaCl cotransporter:*** *Channel protein responsible for reabsorption of sodium and chloride*
- *Drugs that block NaCl cotransporter in DCT—"Thiazide diuretics": Chlorothiazide*
- *Gitelman syndrome is due to mutation in the thiazide sensitive* ***NaCl cotransporter.*** *Its clinical features are hypomagnesemia, hypokalemic metabolic alkalosis, hypocalciuria, hypotension.*
- ***Calcium reabsorption in DCT***
  - *Calcium enters the cell across the apical membrane by a Ca^{++}-permeable ion channel TRPV5.*
  - *It moves out the DCT through Na^{+}/Ca^{++} antiporter present in the basolateral side.*
  - *PTH and Vitamin D act in DCT to increase calcium reabsorption.*

Juxtaglomerular Apparatus

- *Juxtaglomerular apparatus (JGA) refers to the collection of specialized cells seen where DCT touches the glomerulus.*
- *The JGA comprises 3 types of cells namely Juxtaglomerular cells, Macula densa cells and Extraglomerular mesangial cells or Lacis cells.*

  1. ***Juxtaglomerular cells***
     - *They are in the media of the afferent arterioles. They synthesize, store, and release an enzyme called renin. Also called granular cells.*
     - *They release renin whenever there is renal hypoperfusion and hypotension.*
     - *They are densely innervated by the sympathetic nerve fibers—release renin in response to sympathetic discharge.*

2. **Macula densa**
   - These are the specialized epithelial cells of **thick ascending limb of loop of Henle.**
   - They regulate GFR through "Tubuloglomerular feedback".
3. **Extraglomerular mesangial cells:** Also called **"Lacis cells"** or **"Goormaghtigh cells" or "polkissen cells".**

Collecting Duct

- Collecting ducts reabsorb around 4-5% of filtered Na^+.
- Its two important divisions are cortical collecting duct and inner medullary collecting duct.
- Cortical collecting duct is the major site of action of mineralocorticoid hormone "aldosterone". It has two types of cells, namely principal cells (P) and intercalated cells (I).
- Principal cells (P) are the main Na^+-reabsorbing, water reabsorbing and K^+-secreting cells regulated by aldosterone.
- Intercalated cells (I) are of two types namely type A and B intercalated cells. These cells play an important role in acid-base balance.
- **Sodium reabsorption in principal cells**
  - Aldosterone increases sodium resorption by increasing the activity of epithelial sodium channels (ENaCs).
  - Aldosterone prevents degradation of ENaCs by inhibiting Nedd4-2 through SGK1 (**serum and glucocorticoid-regulated kinase 1**).
  - Sodium reabsorption through ENaC is accompanied by water reabsorption that ultimately increases ECF volume.
  - **Epithelial sodium channels (ENaCs) blockers: Diuretics:** Amiloride
  - **Gain of function mutation of Epithelial sodium channels (ENaCs)—"Liddle syndrome":** Severe hypertension with hypokalemia, treatment is ENaC blocker amiloride.
- **Secretion of potassium ion (K^+) in principal cells:** Aldosterone increases the secretion of potassium ion through renal outer medullary potassium (ROMK) channels.
- Water reabsorption in principal cells is under the control of antidiuretic hormone (ADH).

Intercalated Cells

- **Type A intercalated cell** has apical proton pump that mediates acid secretion and basolateral Cl^-/HCO_3^- anion exchanger for bicarbonate reabsorption. kidney preferentially uses type A intercalated cells to secrete the excess H+ under conditions of acidemia.
- Type B looks like the mirror image of type A intercalated cell. kidney preferentially uses type B intercalated cells to secrete the excess HCO_3^- under conditions of alkalemia.

Antidiuretic hormone (ADH) or Vasopressin

- Vasopressin is stored and released from posterior pituitary.
- Herring bodies are the secretory granules of posterior pituitary that contains vasopressin and its precursor peptide **neurophysin.**
- Vasopressin increases water reabsorption in principal cells and inner medullary collecting duct.
- There are three kinds of vasopressin receptors namely $V1_A$ receptor, $V1_B$ receptor, V_2 receptor.
  1. **$V1_A$ receptor:** Vasoconstriction
  2. **V_2 receptor:** Collecting ducts to increase water reabsorption
  3. **$V1_B$ receptor:** Also called V_3 receptor-increases secretion of adrenocorticotropic hormone (ACTH) from anterior pituitary.
- **Antidiuretic effect of vasopressin**
  - Vasopressin acts through V_2 receptors in collecting ducts to increase water reabsorption.
  - It inserts aquaporin 2 into the apical membranes of the principal cells of the collecting ducts for water reabsorption.
- **Factors that increase vasopressin secretion:** Increased effective osmotic pressure of plasma, decreased ECF volume.
- **Factors that decrease vasopressin secretion:** Decreased effective osmotic pressure of plasma, increased ECF volume, alcohol.
- **Vasopressin receptor antagonist (aquaretics):** Conivaptan
- **Obligatory water reabsorption:** Water reabsorption in kidney that is independent of ADH is called obligatory water reabsorption. It mainly happens in the proximal tubules.
- **Facultative water reabsorption:** It is the water reabsorption in kidney under the influence of ADH. It mainly happens in the collecting duct.

FREE WATER CLEARANCE (CH_2O)

- Free water clearance is the amount of solute free water excreted per day.

- Free water clearance will be negative—when concentrated urine is passed due to ADH. Seen in syndrome of inappropriate ADH secretion (SIADH).
- Free water clearance will be positive—when dilute urine is passed in the absence of ADH. Seen in diabetes Insipidus.
- Free water clearance is zero—means kidney lost its concentrating and diluting ability.

NATRIURETIC PEPTIDES

- **Three types:** Atrial natriuretic peptide (ANP), BNP and CNP.
- Increase sodium excretion (natriuresis) by acting in late DCT and collecting duct.
- Renin Angiotensin Aldosterone System (RAAS) and natriuretic peptides system are physiological antagonists.

MICTURITION

- **Innervation of bladder**
  - Parasympathetic supply mainly comes from sacral S2, S3, S4 segments. Also called nervi erigentes. Major function—contraction of detrusor muscle leading to emptying of bladder.
  - Sympathetic supply comes mainly from L1, L2, L3 segments of spinal cord. They are not essential to the act of micturition. Major function—Prevents retrograde ejaculation. They also carry pain information from bladder.
  - Somatic nerve supply: The somatic pudendal nerve (S2, S3 and S4) arises in Onuf's nucleus. It supplies the external sphincter. It is under voluntary control.
- **Higher centers that control micturition**
  - **Pontine micturition center:** Present in the Barrington's nucleus of pons. Facilitates micturition.
  - Posterior hypothalamus—facilitates micturition.
  - Midbrain—inhibits micturition.
  - **Paracentral lobule:** It is supplied by anterior cerebral artery. Lesion in this area causes urinary incontinence.
- **Micturition reflex**
  - Filling of bladder with urine stretches its wall. This stretch information is carried by the sensory afferents fibers in the pelvic nerves to the sacral segments of spinal cord.
  - Parasympathetic fibers to the bladder constitute the efferent limb—it causes the detrusor to contract and relax the internal urethral sphincter eventually leading to micturition.
- Pressure changes associated with bladder filling can be studied with the help of **cystometrogram.**

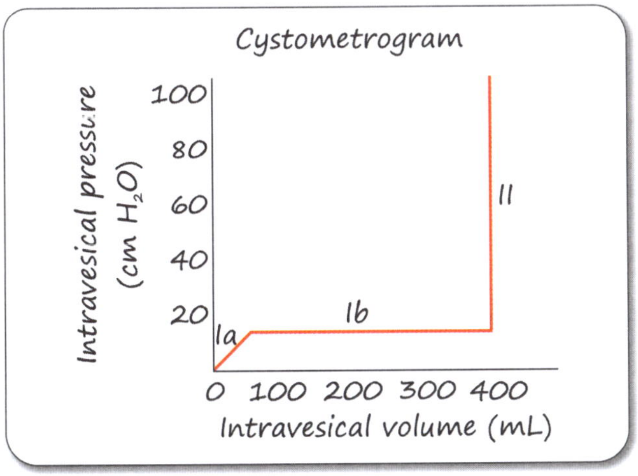

- The graph shows three segments namely Ia, Ib and II
- **Segment Ia**—there is a slight rise in pressure when bladder starts filling
- **Segment Ib**—It's a flat line where bladder is filling with urine but the pressure is not rising. This segment is the manifestation of "**Laplace law**"
- As the urinary bladder gets filled, the tension increases. Since the radius also increases, there is very little increase in pressure according to **Laplace law**
- Segment II—there is a sudden, sharp rise in pressure
- The first urge to void is felt at a bladder volume of about **150 mL**
- Marked sense of fullness—at about **400 mL**

ACID-BASE BALANCE

- Normal pH is 7.35–7.45 (slightly alkaline).
- pH values above 7.80 or below 6.9 are not compatible with life.
- pH changes can denature proteins.
- Low pH (acidosis)—CNS becomes less excitable.
- High pH (alkalosis)—there is hyperexcitability leading to muscle twitches.

Three primary systems regulate the H+ concentration in the body fluids to prevent acidosis or alkalosis:

1. Chemical acid-base buffer system—acts very fast within seconds (First line of defense).
2. The respiratory system—acts in minutes (Second line of defense).
3. Kidneys—acts very slowly (Third line of defense).

1. **Buffers—"The First line of defense"**
   - **Bicarbonate buffer**: The most important extracellular buffer system because the two elements of the buffer system, HCO_3- and CO_2, are regulated precisely by the kidneys and the lungs.
   - Proteins are the most plentiful intracellular buffers in the body.
   - Phosphate buffer is the most important buffer in the tubular fluids of the kidneys.
2. **Respiratory regulation of acid-base balance—"The second line of defense"**
   - An increase in ventilation eliminates CO_2 from extracellular fluid: During acidosis
   - Decreased ventilation increases CO_2: During alkalosis
   - The feedback gain for respiratory regulation of acid-base balance is around 3 (only 75% effective).
3. **Renal regulation of acid-base balance—"The third line of defense"**
   - Helps in reabsorption of filtered HCO_3^-
   - **Generation of new HCO_3^-**: Phosphate buffer and ammonia buffer are utilized to neutralize acid in place of bicarbonate buffer.
   - **Excretion of acid:** During acidosis using Type A intercalated cells.
   - **Excretion of HCO_3^-**: During alkalosis using Type B intercalated cells.

MUST KNOW

- H^+ ions are secreted into the urine till urinary pH reaches 4.5. This pH of 4.5 is termed the limiting pH.
- Limiting pH is reached only in collecting tubule. Acidification of urine happens in collecting duct.

Normal values	pH	H^+	PCO_2	HCO_3^-
	7.4	40 nanomoles/L	40 mm Hg	24 mEq/L

Metabolic acidosis

- Primary problem in metabolic acidosis is loss of HCO_3^- or addition of nonvolatile acids causing decrease in pH.
- Important causes of metabolic acidosis are diabetic ketoacidosis, lactic acidosis and vomiting of intestinal contents (loss of bicarbonate).
- **Anion gap:** Refers to those anions which are present but are not determined routinely. Mainly due to plasma protein anions, sulfate and phosphate. Normal anion gap value is between 8 and 16 mEq/L.
- **Normochloremic metabolic acidosis:** To maintain electroneutrality, the concentration of unmeasured anion rises: it is called normochloremic metabolic acidosis or high anion gap metabolic acidosis (HAGMA).
- Important causes of HAGMA are diabetic ketoacidosis, lactic acidosis, salicylic acid poisoning and ethylene glycol poisoning.
- **Hyperchloremic metabolic acidosis:** To maintain electroneutrality, here chloride ion increases: this condition is called normal anion gap metabolic acidosis (NAGMA).
- Important causes of NAGMA are renal tubular acidosis, diarrhea and hypoaldosteronism.
- **Compensations seen in metabolic acidosis:** Respiratory compensation—hyperventilation and renal compensation—Increased expression of type A intercalated cells that secrete H^+ in urine.

Metabolic alkalosis

- Primary problem in metabolic acidosis is loss of H^+ or addition of HCO_3^- causing increase in pH.
- Causes of metabolic alkalosis are vomiting of gastric contents (loss of H^+), hyperaldosteronism (loss of H^+ in urine), excessive ingestion of antacids, volume contraction alkalosis—administration of thiazide diuretics.

- **Compensations seen in metabolic alkalosis:** Respiratory compensation—Hypoventilation and renal compensation—Increased expression of type B intercalated cells that secrete HCO_3^- in urine.

Respiratory Acidosis

- Primary problem in respiratory acidosis is increased pCO_2 that causes an increase in H^+ and lowering of blood pH.
- Causes are depression of respiratory center by drugs like opioids, damage to respiratory centers, weakening of respiratory muscles – polio, Guillain-Barre syndrome, Impaired gas diffusion – COPD
- Compensation is mainly renal: Increased reabsorption of new HCO_3^- and excretion of acid.

Respiratory Alkalosis

- Primary problem in respiratory alkalosis is decreased pCO_2 that causes a decrease in H+ and increase in blood pH.
- Seen in individuals who ascend to high altitude, psychogenic hyperventilation.
- Compensation is mainly renal which includes increased expression of type B intercalated cells that secrete HCO_3^- in urine.

Notes

9. GASTROINTESTINAL PHYSIOLOGY

FUNCTIONS AND STRUCTURAL CHARACTERISTICS OF GASTROINTESTINAL TRACT

- Two major functions of the gastrointestinal (GI) tract are **Secretion** of juices rich in enzymes that aid in digestion of food substances and **Motility** function that moves food particles across various segments of GI tract for digestion and absorption.
- To regulate these functions, GI tract is well equipped with **Enteric nervous system and GI hormones.**

Structural characteristics of GI Tract

- **Serosa:** Outermost layer
- **Muscular layer:** Circular muscle layer and longitudinal muscle layer. **Auerbach nerve plexus** (also called myenteric plexus) is present in between circular and longitudinal muscle fibers. This plexus is concerned primarily with motor control (Myenteric: Motility).
- **Submucosa:** Contains blood vessels, lymphatics and a nerve plexus called Meissner's plexus (submucosal plexus). This plexus is primarily involved in the control of intestinal secretion (Submucosal: Secretion and blood flow).
- **Mucosa:** Innermost layer. Contains muscularis mucosa that contracts and alters the available surface of GI tract.

GASTROINTESTINAL SECRETIONS

MUST KNOW

- Human intestines are presented with 9000 mL of fluid every day (2000 mL ingested fluid plus 7000 mL endogenous GI secretions).
- Out of this 9000 mL of fluid, around 8800 mL of fluid is effectively reabsorbed (98%). The remaining 200 mL is excreted in stool.

Salivary secretion:

- Total salivary secretion- 1500 mL/day
- pH of saliva is 6–7.
- Saliva is hypotonic to plasma.
- Comes from three major salivary glands namely **Submandibular gland, Parotid gland and Sublingual gland.**
- **Minor salivary glands:** Superior pole of tonsils **(Weber glands)**, base of tongue **(von Ebner glands)**
- **Digestive enzymes present in saliva:** Salivary amylase (ptyalin) for carbohydrate digestion. Lingual lipase for lipid digestion produced by Ebner's gland.
- Saliva contains anti-bacterial substances like lysozyme and Lactoferrin. It also contains **immunoglobulin A** (IgA).
- Saliva also contains the blood group substances A, B, AB and O.
- Acinar cells—secrete primary salivary secretion.
- Ductal secretion—modifies the primary secretion by reabsorbing Na^+, Cl^- and secreting potassium (K^+) and bicarbonate ions (HCO_3^-) – "Hypotonic saliva"
- Both sympathetic and parasympathetic increase salivary secretion with parasympathetic having greater influence.
- Glossopharyngeal nerve through otic ganglion innervates **Parotid gland.**
- Facial nerve through submandibular ganglion innervates Submandibular gland and Sublingual gland.

Gastric Secretion

- Gastric secretion is the maximum amount of secretion that is secreted every day in GI tract—It is 2500 mL. It is also the highly acidic GI secretion—pH is <3.
- **Cells of the gastric mucosa:**
  - **Surface cells:** Produce mucus.
  - **Mucus neck cells:** Stem cells.
  - **Parietal cells:** Involved in gastric acid secretion and intrinsic factor for Vitamin B_{12} absorption.
  - **Enterochromaffin like cells (ECL cells):** Produce histamine.
  - **Chief cells:** Produce pepsinogen.
- **Pepsinogen is converted to pepsin by gastric acid.** Pepsin helps in protein digestion. Gastric lipase helps in lipid digestion.
- **Parietal cells:** H^+, K^+-ATPase, or proton pump that pump H^+ into the lumen against a concentration gradient.
- Bicarbonate is pumped out of the parietal cell in change for chloride ions using a chloride-bicarbonate exchanger.

- Chloride ions (Cl^-) in parietal cells are pumped out from the apical side into the lumen through a chloride channel (ClC). In the lumen, H^+ ions react with Cl^- ions to form HCl (gastric acid).
- The HCO_3^- released into the blood is responsible for **post-prandial alkaline tide—seen after meals.**
- Three major factors that increase gastric acid secretion are:
  - Histamine—paracrine factor (released from a nearby ECL cell).
  - Gastrin—Endocrine factor (Released by G cells into blood that reaches parietal cells).
  - Acetylcholine—neurocrine factor (released by vagal nerve endings).
- **Histamine acts through** H_2 receptor. **Gastrin** acts through CCK-B receptors and **Acetylcholine (ACH)** acts through M_3 receptors.
- **Factors that decrease gastric acid secretion:**
  - Gastric acid itself—negative feedback mechanism
  - Somatostatin
  - Gastric inhibitory peptide (GIP)
  - Prostaglandins
- Gastric secretion occurs in three different phases namely Cephalic phase, Gastric phase and Intestinal phase.
  - **Cephalic phase:** Accounts for 30% of gastric secretion. The secretion is initiated by the thought, sight, smell, or taste of food.
  - **Gastric phase:** Accounts for 60% of gastric secretion. Activated when food enters the stomach.
  - **Intestinal phase:** Accounts for 10% of gastric secretion. Activated when chyme enters the duodenum.
- **Zollinger–Ellison syndrome (ZES):** Characterized by gastric acid hypersecretion due to tumor (gastrinoma). Peptic ulcer is the most common clinical manifestation. Such ulcers are refractory to standard medical therapy and they recur after acid-reducing surgery. Proton pump inhibitors are the treatment of choice for ZES.
- **Pernicious anemia:** Autoimmune disease. Auto antibodies destroy Parietal cells. Characterized by **achlorhydria, reduced secretion of pepsin** from stomach and increased serum levels of gastrin.

Exocrine Pancreatic Secretion

- About 1500 mL of pancreatic juice is secreted per day. It is alkaline with pH 7.8–8.4 with very high concentration of bicarbonate.
- Most of the pancreatic enzymes are stored as inactive forms (zymogens). This is mainly to prevent the **autodigestion** of pancreas.
- Trypsinogen is converted to the active form trypsin in intestine by enterokinase.
- Once formed, trypsin activates all the other pancreatic enzymes to their active forms in intestine.
- Pancreatic α-amylase helps in carbohydrate digestion. Pancreatic lipase and colipase help in lipid digestion. Trypsin, Chymotrypsin and Carboxypeptidase help in protein digestion.
- Bicarbonate is secreted into lumen in exchange for chloride ion. This bicarbonate ion makes pancreatic secretion highly alkaline.
- Movement of chloride into lumen is by cystic fibrosis transmembrane conductance regulator (CFTR). Mutations in CFTR gene cause **cystic fibrosis.**
- Two major hormones that regulate pancreatic secretion are cholecystokinin and secretin.

Secretin	Cholecystokinin – Pancreozymin (CCK-PZ)
• Acidic chyme releases Secretin. • It acts on the pancreatic ducts. • It causes alkaline pancreatic juice that **is rich in HCO_3^-** and poor in enzymes • It neutralizes the gastric acid—referred to as "nature's antacid" • Second messenger: cAMP	• Fats and amino acids release CCK. • It acts on the acinar cells. • It causes the release of zymogen granules and production of pancreatic juice **rich in enzymes** but low in volume. • Action is mediated by phospholipase C.

Biliary Secretion

- About 500 mL of bile is secreted per day.
- **Gallbladder:** Storage of bile and concentration of bile.
- Bile acids are the major components of bile. The two primary bile acids are cholic acid and chenodeoxycholic acid.
- In the intestine, they are dehydroxylated by bacteria to form secondary bile acids which are deoxycholic acid and lithocholic acid.
- In the liver, bile acids are conjugated with glycine or taurine to form the conjugated bile acids glycocholic acid and taurocholic acid.

- **Bile salts:** Conjugated bile acids combine with sodium or potassium ions to form the salts.
- **Enterohepatic circulation:** In intestine, bile acids are absorbed actively in ileum using Na^+-dependent transport proteins and travel through the portal blood to the liver, where they are taken up by the hepatocytes and resecreted. This process happens 6 to 8 times per day and it helps in conserving energy needed to produce bile salts.
- **Bile helps in digestion and absorption of fat by forming** cylindrical disks called **micelles.**
- Substances excreted in bile are bile pigments, heavy metals, toxins and cholesterol.
- **Choleretics:** Substances that enhance secretion of bile salts. Example: Bile salts
- **Cholagogues:** Substances that cause contraction of gallbladder. Example: **Cholecystokinin (CCK).**

Small Intestinal Secretions

- Intestinal juice is also called succus entericus. It contains enterokinase which activates trypsinogen to trypsin.
- It is secreted by the cells present in the crypts of Lieberkühn.
- Crypts of lieberkühn contain three types of cells namely goblet cells (secrete mucus), Epithelial cells and Paneth cells.
- Paneth cells are present in the base of crypts. They have high concentration of Zinc. They secrete defensins—an antimicrobial peptide. They also secrete lysozymes.

GASTROINTESTINAL HORMONES

Gastrointestinal (GI) hormones are classified into gastrin family, Secretin family and others.

1. **Gastrin family:** Gastrin, Cholecystokinin.
2. **Secretin family:** Secretin, gastrin inhibitory peptide (GIP), glucagon like peptide (GLP), vasoactive intestinal peptide (VIP).
3. **Others:** Motilin, Guanylin, peptide YY, ghrelin.

Enteroendocrine cell	Secreting hormone
G cells	Gastrin
I cells	Cholecystokinin
S cells	Secretin
K cells	Gastric inhibitory peptide or glucose-dependent insulinotropic peptide (GIP)
Mo cells	Motilin
D cells	Somatostatin

GI hormone	Characteristics
Gastrin	• Produced by G cells in the antral portion of the gastric mucosa. G 17 is the principal form. • Peptides, amino acids, gastric distension and gastrin releasing peptide increase gastrin secretion. • Acid, somatostatin, Secretin and GIP inhibit gastrin secretion. • Acts via CCK-B receptor. • Actions: Stimulation of gastric acid secretion, stimulation of the growth of the mucosa of GI tract (trophic action).
Cholecystokinin (CCK)	• Secreted by I cells in the mucosa of the upper small intestine. • Acts via CCK-A receptor. • Peptides and amino acids, fatty acids increase CCK secretion. • **Functions in gut:** Stimulation of pancreatic enzyme secretion, contraction of the gallbladder. • **Functions in brain:** Regulation of food intake, anxiety and analgesia. • **Other actions:** Augments the action of secretin, inhibits gastric emptying, exerts a trophic effect on the pancreas.

Contd...

GI hormone	Characteristics
Secretin	• First hormone identified by Bayliss and Starling. • Secreted by S cells (mucosa of the upper portion of the small intestine). • Increases secretion of bicarbonate by duct cells of pancreas. • Augments the action of CCK, decreases gastric acid secretion. • Stimulus that increases secretin secretion is acidic chyme.
Gastric inhibitory peptide (GIP)	• Produced by K cells. • Secretion is stimulated by glucose and fat in the duodenum. • Stimulates insulin secretion—called glucose-dependent insulinotropic peptide (GIP). • Glucagon like peptide (GLP) and gastric inhibitory peptide (GIP) are called Incretins that increase insulin secretion.
Vasoactive intestinal peptide (VIP)	• Stimulates intestinal secretion of electrolytes and water, and relaxes intestinal smooth muscles. • potentiates the action of acetylcholine in salivary glands.
Motilin	• Secreted by Mo cells. • Contracts smooth muscles in the stomach and intestines in between meals- Migratory Motor Complex.
Guanylin	• Causes increased secretion of Cl^- into the intestinal lumen. • E. coli has a structure very similar to guanylin and activates guanylin receptors in the intestine (Molecular Mimicry).
Peptide YY	• Stimulated by the presence of fat. • Ileal brake: When lipids or carbohydrates are infused into the ileum, there is Inhibition of gastric and pancreatic secretion and motility. Peptide YY is responsible for ileal brake.
Ghrelin	• Secreted primarily by oxyntic gland area of the stomach. • It increases the appetite (orexinergic). • Increases gastric motility and secretion of gastric acid. • Increases growth hormone. • Ghrelin levels peak just before food intake begins (fasting state). • Plasma levels of ghrelin are low in obese persons. • Ghrelin levels are high in anorexia nervosa.

REGULATION OF FOOD INTAKE

- Agents that increase food intake are called **orexigenic substances or appetite stimulants**. They are Neuropeptide Y (NPY), Agouti-related protein (AGRP) and Ghrelin.
- Agents that decrease food intake are called **anorexigenic substances or satiety promoting factors**. They are Melanocyte-stimulating hormone (α-MSH), Cocaine- and amphetamine-regulated transcript (CART), Leptin, Insulin and Cholecystokinin (CCK).

DIGESTION AND ABSORPTION

Carbohydrates

- In mouth, saliva contains salivary amylase or ptyalin for digestion of carbohydrates. In stomach, there is no enzyme for carbohydrate digestion. In exocrine pancreas, pancreatic amylase hydrolyzes α ($1 \rightarrow 4$) glycoside bonds of starch. In small intestine, Brush border enzymes namely disaccharidases like maltase converts maltose to glucose and Lactase—converts lactose to glucose and galactose.

- Carbohydrates are absorbed mainly from duodenum and jejunum.
- **Glucose and galactose:** Absorbed by a sodium-dependent process—SGLT 1. This type of transport is an example of secondary active transport.
- Fructose is absorbed from intestinal lumen into the enterocytes by **GLUT5**.
- Congenital absence of SGLT-1 leads to **congenital glucose galactose malabsorption** (CGGM).

Lipids

- In mouth, saliva contains lingual lipase for digestion of lipids. In stomach, gastric lipase is present. In exocrine pancreas, Pancreatic lipase—splits triglycerides to fatty acids and monoglycerides. Colipase—aids the function of lipase.
- Lipids are absorbed mainly from duodenum and jejunum.
- Fatty acids are emulsified by bile salts. They are transported to the brush border cells using micelles. Once inside the enterocytes, they are resynthesized to triglycerides and packed into chylomicrons by enterocytes and transported.
- Lipid absorption is by simple diffusion (passive process).

Proteins

- In mouth, there are no enzymes for protein digestion. In stomach, Pepsin cleaves peptide bonds. In exocrine pancreas, Trypsin, Chymotrypsin and Carboxypeptidase digest dietary proteins to dipeptides and tripeptides.
- Dipeptides and tripeptides—transported into enterocytes using PepT1 (peptide transporter 1). Inside enterocytes, cytoplasmic proteases act on them and convert them into amino acids.
- Amino acids are transported into the blood vessels using basolateral amino acid transporters.

Vitamins

- Fat soluble vitamins A, D, E, K are absorbed dissolved in the lipid micelles.
- Except Vitamin B_{12} and folate, all the other water-soluble vitamins require sodium for their absorption. Vitamin B_{12} is absorbed in the ileum.

ABSORPTION OF IRON

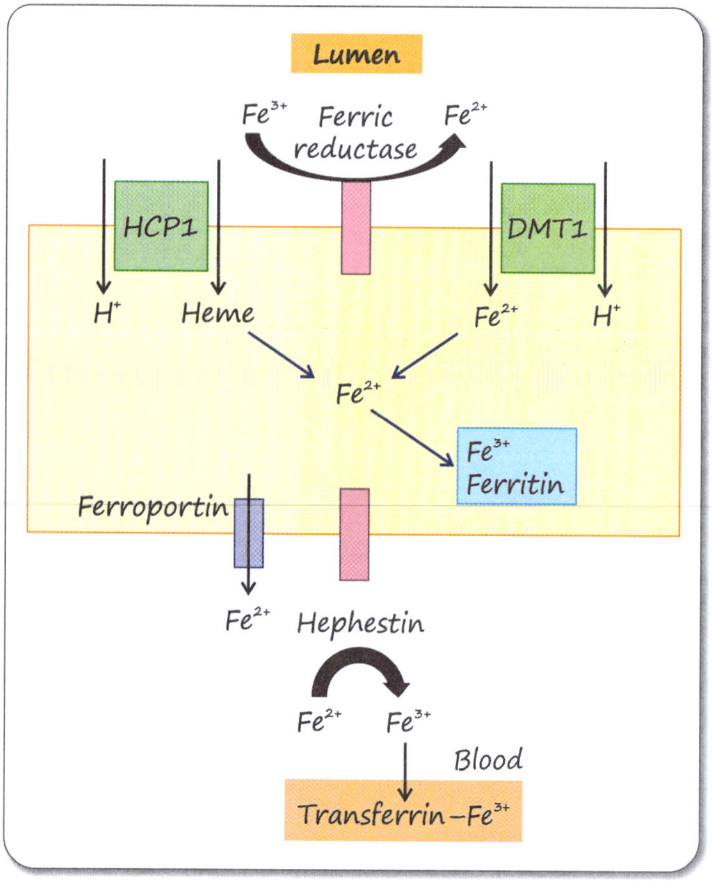

- Absorption of iron mainly occurs in duodenum.
- Fe^{3+} (ferric) is converted to Fe^{2+} (ferrous) by the ferric reductase DCYTB.
- Fe^{2+} is transported into the enterocyte by the apical membrane iron transporter DMT1.
- Heme is transported into the enterocyte by heme transporter heme carrier protein 1, HCP1.
- Intracellular Fe^{2+} is converted to Fe^{3+} and stored as ferritin.
- Basolateral Fe^{2+} transporter ferroportin-1 (FPN1) transports Fe^{2+} out
- The transport is aided by hephaestin (Heph) which converts Fe^{2+} to Fe^{3+}.
- In plasma, Fe^{3+} is transported bound to the iron transport protein transferrin (TF).

MUST KNOW

Hepcidin

- Hepcidin is produced by the liver. It represses the basolateral transport of iron into blood by binding to **ferroportin.**
- Its level is regulated by HFE gene. Mutations in HFE gene—hemochromatosis.

GASTROINTESTINAL MOTILITY

- Type of muscles present in GI tract is single unit smooth muscle with gap junctions.
- **Pacemakers of GI tract—"Interstitial cells of Cajal".** They are mainly responsible for the **"generation of basic electrical rhythm (BER)".**
- **Pacemaker cells in stomach are in the midbody of the stomach along the greater curvature.**
- The oscillating membrane potential between -60 and -40 mV in GI smooth muscles is termed **basic electrical rhythm (BER).** BER is also called "slow waves". **Rate of BER in duodenum is highest** (12/min) and in cecum, it is lowest (2/min).
- **Acetylcholine increases** the number of spikes and the tension of the smooth muscle, whereas **epinephrine decreases** the number of spikes and tension.
- **Deglutition (swallowing)**
  - It comprises three stages namely oral phase—voluntary, Pharyngeal phase—involuntary, Esophageal phase—involuntary.
  - Afferent for deglutition reflex is 5th, 9th and 10th cranial nerves. Center is nucleus tractus solitarius in medulla. Efferent is cranial nerves 5, 7 and hypoglossal nerve.
- **Motility events in the esophagus**
  - Food bolus is pushed from esophagus to the stomach by peristalsis.
  - Primary stimulus that initiates peristalsis is the stretch.
  - Peristalsis has two segments: Contracting segment and Relaxing segment.
    1. **Contracting segment behind the bolus:** Neurotransmitters responsible are substance P and acetylcholine.
    2. **Relaxing segment in front of the bolus:** Neurotransmitters responsible are nitric oxide and vasoactive intestinal peptide.
  - Three types of peristalsis seen in esophagus are as follows:
    1. **Primary peristalsis:** Progressive, physiological.
    2. **Secondary peristalsis:** Progressive, seen during irritation of esophagus.
    3. **Tertiary peristalsis:** Nonprogressive-responsible for esophageal spasm.
  - **Achalasia cardia:** Lower esophageal sphincter (LES) fails to relax in response to deglutition—it is a state of tonic contraction. There is deficient myenteric plexus of the esophagus at the LES in this condition and the release of nitric oxide. Treated with injections of botulinum toxin (Botox) directly into the LES—blocks acetylcholine release that prevents smooth muscle contraction.
- **Gastric motility**
  - Stomach aids in storage of food and mixing and grinding of ingested solid food particles.
  - **Receptive relaxation:** Seen in proximal stomach—aids in accommodation of the incoming food termed gastric accommodation.
  - **Retropulsion:** Stomach forces food particles to be propelled against a closed pylorus. Since the pylorus is closed, there is **retropulsion** of solids and liquids back into the stomach. This helps in mixing and grinding of ingested food particles.
  - Gastric emptying is fastest for foods rich in carbohydrate. It is slow for protein rich diet and is slowest for fat rich diet.
  - Gastrin and increased food volume in the stomach **increase gastric emptying.**
  - Factors that inhibit gastric emptying:
    - **Fats, carbohydrates and acid in the duodenum:** Initiates enterogastric reflex, a type of enteric reflex which decreases gastric emptying.
    - Hyperosmolality of the duodenal contents.
    - Cholecystokinin.
  - **Defecation following a meal in newborn:** Gastrocolic reflex. This reflex is amplified by gastrin.
- **Movements of small intestine**
  - **Segmentation contractions:** Segment of bowel contracts at both ends that retard the food movement. Provides adequate time for mixing of food with digestive juices.
  - Peristalsis
- **Movements of large intestine**
  - **Proximal colon:** Mainly for absorption of water and electrolytes.
  - **Distal colon:** Mainly for storage of feces.

  - **Haustrations:** Combined contractions of the circular and longitudinal muscles of colon.
  - **Mass movements:** Contractions move colonic contents from one segment of colon to another. Initiates **defecation reflex.**
- **Defecation**
  - Defecation is the process of excretion of fecal material.
  - **Internal anal sphincter:** Formed by thickened circular smooth muscle. It is involuntary. It is relaxed by parasympathetic nerve fibers—facilitates defecation.
  - **External anal sphincter:** Formed by skeletal muscle (somatic). It is voluntary and innervated by pudendal nerve.
  - Distension of the rectum with feces initiates defecation reflex. Afferent impulses pass through the pelvic nerves to sacral spinal segment.
  - In response to that, there is reflex parasympathetic discharge that causes relaxation of internal anal sphincter. Simultaneously, voluntary relaxation of external sphincter occurs leading to defecation.
  - The urge to defecate first occurs—when rectal pressure increases to about 18 mm Hg.
  - When this pressure reaches 55 mm Hg—there is relaxation of internal and external anal sphincters leading to reflex expulsion of feces.

COLONIC FLORA

- Ferment dietary starches to form Short-chain fatty acids (SCFAs).
- SCFAs are acetate, propionate and butyrate. These fatty acids are the principal source of nutrition for the colonocyte. They are absorbed in part by exchange for H^+, helping maintain acid-base equilibrium.

Migratory Motor Complex

- Migratory motor complex (MMC) is the predominant motility pattern seen during fasting state.
- Occurs at intervals of approximately 90-100 minutes in the interdigestive state. Initiated by motilin.
- Aids in clearing the stomach and small intestine of luminal contents in preparation for the next meal.
- Erythromycin-binds to motilin receptors. Useful in treating patients with reduced GI motility.

DIETARY FIBERS

- Also called roughage.
- **Examples:** Cellulose, Hemicellulose, Lignin, Pectins
- **Importance of dietary fibers**
  - Add bulk to the diet—may reduce appetite.
  - Slow the absorption of glucose.
  - Lower total and LDL cholesterol.
  - Decrease transit time of food in GIT.
  - Water soluble fibers are fermented by microflora to form short-chain fatty acids.
  - They are hydrophilic, thereby leading to water reabsorption and stool bulking.
  - They prevent the formation of colonic diverticula.

10. EXERCISE PHYSIOLOGY

TYPES OF EXERCISES AND SOURCES OF ENERGY FOR MUSCLES

- Other than offering enormous health benefits, exercise is employed therapeutically in the treatment of diabetes mellitus and other related disorders.
- Two types of exercises are there, namely Isotonic exercise and Isometric exercise.
  - **Isotonic exercise:** Also called "dynamic exercise." Tension generated in the muscle is constant. Length of the muscle changes. Example: Treadmill running.
  - **Isometric exercise:** Also called "static exercise". Tension generated in the muscle increases. Length of the muscle does not change. Example: Push against the wall.
- Three important sources supply energy for the exercising muscle. They are Phosphocreatine system, Glycogen-lactic acid system and Aerobic system.
  1. The energy released by Phosphocreatine system can sustain exercise for **8–10 seconds.** For example, 100-meter run.
  2. Glycogen-lactic acid system provides energy to sustain activity up to **1.3–1.6 minutes.**
  3. Aerobic system provides energy during prolonged activities like long distance running (endurance type).

CARDIOVASCULAR RESPONSES TO EXERCISE

- Increase in skeletal muscle blood flow
  - At rest, skeletal muscle receives 2–4 mL/100 g/min. But during exercise, the value increases by >20 times – 80 mL/100 g/min.
  - This increase is mainly because of accumulation of local metabolites that cause vasodilation.
- Redistribution of blood flow in the body
  - Blood flow to renal circulation and splanchnic blood flow decreases.
  - Coronary blood flow increases.
  - Cutaneous blood flow initially decreases, later increases.
  - Cerebral blood flow remains largely unchanged.
- Increase in cardiac output
  - Increase in heart rate which is responsible for most of the increase in cardiac output.
  - Heart rate rises even before the start of exercise- termed **anticipatory tachycardia:** due to psychic stimuli and afferent impulses from proprioceptors in muscles, tendons and joints.
- Blood pressure changes
  - During isotonic exercise, systolic BP rises, and diastolic pressure usually remains unchanged or falls. In exercising muscle, there is accumulation of local metabolites leading to vasodilation—this causes decrease in peripheral resistance leading to fall in diastolic pressure.
  - During isometric exercise, both systolic and diastolic BP rise. Since the exercising muscle is tonically contracted—there is increase in total peripheral resistance and increase in diastolic pressure.

RESPIRATORY RESPONSES TO EXERCISE

- Increase in pulmonary ventilation: Exercise increases the plasma K^+ level that stimulates peripheral chemoreceptors: This stimulates respiration during exercise.
- Increase in respiratory rate that occurs abruptly at the start of exercise is termed anticipatory tachypnea.
- **Increase in oxygen uptake**
  - **VO_2 max:** Highest oxygen uptake achieved during exercise.
  - **Peak VO_2:** If a person stops doing exercise prematurely due to cardiorespiratory limitations—the highest oxygen uptake by that individual at the end of the test is called Peak VO_2. It may not be same as the VO_2 max.
  - **Metabolic equivalent (MET):** One MET is equivalent to the resting oxygen consumption; for an average man—it is 250 mL/min and for woman, it is 200 mL/ min.
  - **Excess post-exercise oxygen consumption (EPOC):** Increase in oxygen consumption post exercise.
- During exercise, arterial pH, PCO_2 and PO_2 remain constant.

REGULATION OF BODY TEMPERATURE

- Normal body temperature: 36.8 ± 0.4°C or 98.2 ± 0.7°F

- **Body temperature—circadian rhythm:** Lowest in morning and highest in the evening.
- Temperature sensors in human body are transient receptor potential (TRP) channels.
- **Heat sensing:** $TRPV_1$, $TRPM_2$, M_3 and $TRPA_1$
- **Cold sensing:** $TRPM_8$
- **Unit of heat measurement: Calorie:** It is the amount of heat required to raise the temperature of 1 g of water by 1°C.
- Metabolism in human body is an important source of heat generation.
- Respiratory quotient (RQ) is the volume of CO_2 produced divided by the volume of O_2 consumed.
- **RQ values:** Carbohydrates is 1, Proteins is 0.8, Fats is 0.7 and Mixed diet is 0.82
- Evaporation, conduction, convection and radiation are important sources of heat loss.
- **Anterior hypothalamus:** Activated by hot temperature. Activation causes cutaneous vasodilation, sweating and increase in thirst sensation (osmoreceptors are present in anterior hypothalamus).
- **Posterior Hypothalamus:** Activated by cold temperature. Activation causes shivering, vasoconstriction and increase in urinary frequency.
- **Feed forward control or Anticipatory control:** Temperature control—thermoregulatory responses are initiated by hypothalamus before the changes in environmental temperature have succeeded in changing the body's core body temperature.
- **Fever:** change in hypothalamic set point caused by pyrogens.
- **Prostaglandin E_2:** Acts on EP_3 receptors: alteration of hypothalamic set point-fever.

Heat Disorders Along with their Characteristics

Name	Characteristics
Heat Cramps	• Mild heat disorder • Due to working in hot environment • Thermoregulatory mechanisms intact • Treatment-electrolyte replacement fluid
Heat Syncope	• Mild heat disorder • Caused by prolonged standing in hot environment • Thermoregulatory mechanisms intact • Reduced diastolic filling to heart—reduced cardiac output—reduced cerebral blood flow- syncopal attacks • Treatment-recovery by lying down
Heat Exhaustion	• Excessive vasodilation-reduced diastolic filling to heart • Also called heat collapse • Thermoregulatory mechanisms intact • Treatment-recovery by lying down and fluid replacement
Heat Stroke	• Severe heat disorder-medical emergency • Thermoregulatory mechanisms NOT intact • No sweating • Treatment- cold water bath, cold clothes, fluid replacement
Malignant Hyperthermia	• Due to mutations in ryanodine receptor • This mutation releases excess calcium from sarcoplasmic reticulum leading to excessive muscle contraction and increased body temperature • Triggered by neuromuscular blocking drug succinylcholine • Usually treated using ryanodine receptor blocker **dantrolene**

Hypothermia

- **Accidental causes:** Exposure to cold environment, drugs like barbiturates.
- **Therapeutic hypothermia:** For every 1°C fall in body temperature, cerebral blood flow decreases by 7%.
- Therapeutic hypothermia is useful during neurosurgical procedures to minimize blood loss.
- **Cardiomyocyte cooling:** In acute myocardial infarction—return of spontaneous circulation (ROSC) can lead to death because of oxidative stress. To prevent this, cardiomyocyte cooling is done.

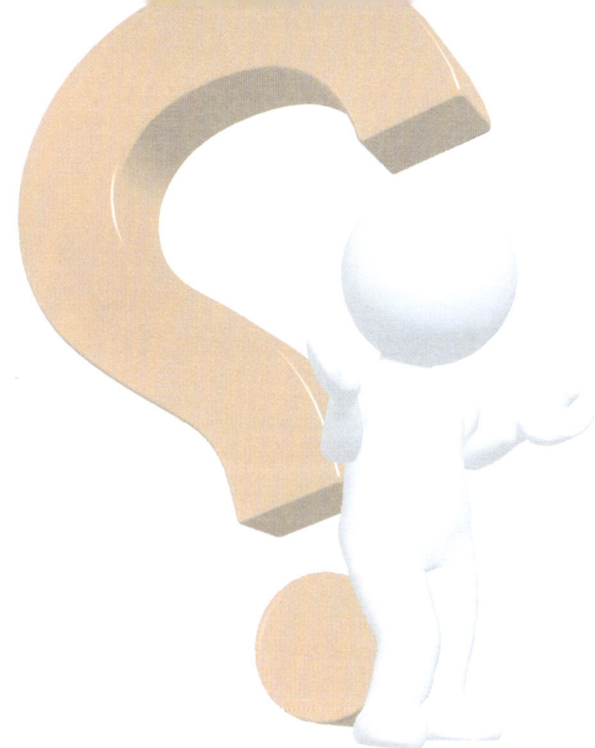

Latest Question Papers

- → NEET PG 2023
- → NEET PG 2022
- → NEET PG 2021
- → INI-CET NOVEMBER 2023
- → INI-CET MAY 2023
- → INI-CET NOVEMBER 2022
- → INI-CET MAY 2022
- → INI-CET NOVEMBER 2021
- → INI-CET JULY 2021
- → FMGE JANUARY 2024
- → FMGE JANUARY 2023
- → FMGE JULY 2023
- → FMGE JUNE 2022
- → FMGE DECEMBER 2021
- → FMGE JUNE 2021

NEET PG 2023

1. **Which of the following statement is true regarding myocardial action potential curve?**
   a. Due to slow but prolonged opening of Ca^{2+} channels—Phase 2
   b. Open Na and close fast K channels—Phase 4
   c. Close Na channel and open slow K channel—Phase 0
   d. Is due to Na^+/K^+ ATPase- Phase 3

Ans. a. Due to slow but prolonged opening of Ca^{2+} channels—Phase 2

2. **Carrier protein mediated transport across the cell membrane is:**
   a. Primary active transport
   b. Simple diffusion
   c. Facilitated diffusion
   d. Secondary active transport

Ans. c. Facilitated diffusion

3. **Functional residual capacity includes:**
   a. Tidal volume and inspiratory reserve volume
   b. Inspiratory reserve volume and expiratory reserve volume
   c. Inspiratory reserve volume and residual volume
   d. Residual volume and expiratory reserve volume

Ans. d. Residual volume and expiratory reserve volume

4. **A preterm baby was delivered at 28 weeks. Which of the following is true about surface tension compliance?**
   a. Surface tension increases; compliance decreases
   b. Surface tension decreases; compliance increases
   c. Both decrease
   d. Both increase

Ans. a. Surface tension increases; compliance decreases

5. **The respective substances in the clearance graph are:**

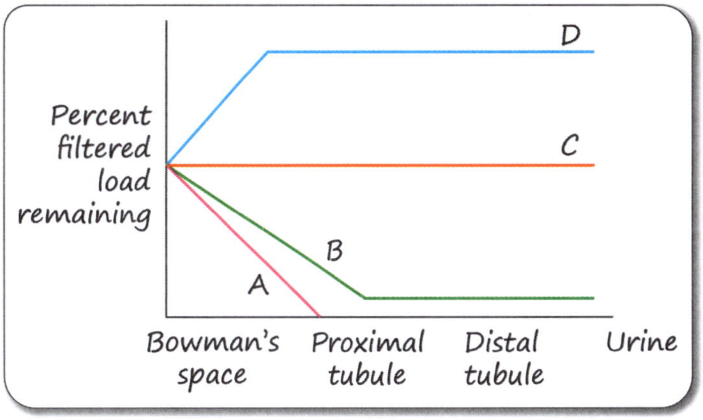

   a. A- inulin; B- Glucose; C- PAH; D- Bicarbonate
   b. A- Glucose; B- Bicarbonate; C- inulin; D- PAH
   c. A- inulin; B- Bicarbonate; C- PAH; D- Glucose
   d. A- PAH; B- Glucose; C- PAH; D- Inulin

Ans. b. A- Glucose; B-Bicarbonate; C- Inulin; D-PAH

6. **A person came to the hospital after RTI. He had severe muscle injury. Serum K^+ level was 5.5 mEq. What would happen to RMP?**
   a. No change
   b. More positive
   c. More negative
   d. First positive, then negative

Ans. b. More positive

7. **Penetrating cervical neck trauma is piercing the lateral aspect of dorsal column tract. Which of the following finding is seen?**
   a. Absence of ipsilateral proprioception of arm
   b. Absence of ipsilateral proprioception of lower limb
   c. Absence of fine motor movement of fingers
   d. Absence of contralateral proprioception of lower limb

Ans. a. Absence of ipsilateral proprioception of arm

8. A laborer becomes unconscious and is brought to ER with temperature of 105°F and decreased skin turgor. Which of the following is not seen in the patient?

a. Tachypnea
b. Hypotension
c. Sweating
d. Red hot skin

Ans. c. Sweating

NEET PG 2022

9. A patient whose hypothalamic thermostat was reset from A to C. What happens in stage B compared to A?

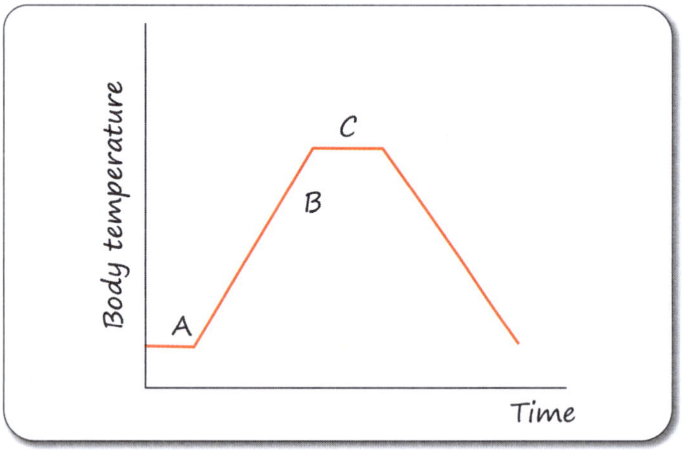

a. Shivering
b. Sweating
c. Increased blood flow to skin
d. Inhibition of chemical thermogenesis

Ans. a. Shivering

10. Blood pressure regulation by baroreceptors is an example of:

a. Feed forward
b. Positive feedback
c. Negative feedback
d. Adaptive control regulation

Ans. c. Negative feedback

11. A patient suffering from stroke presents on the 2nd day with the flailing of limbs. The lesion is present in which of the following structures?

a. Subthalamic nuclei
b. Globus pallidus
c. Putamen
d. Caudate

Ans. a. Subthalamic nuclei

12. Which of the following statement is correct regarding cystometrogram?

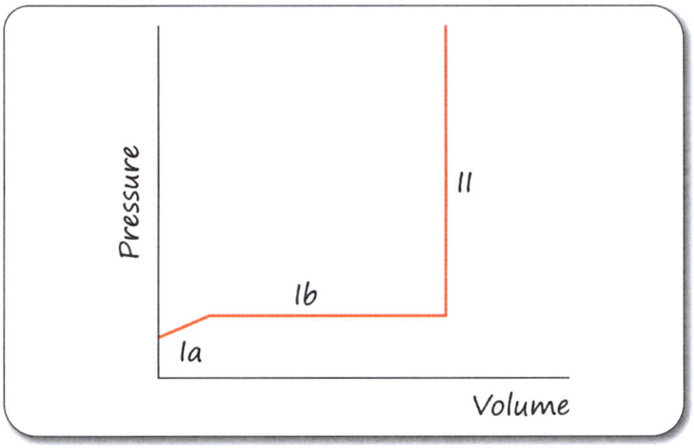

a. Ia is due to residual urine
b. Ib is due to Laplace law
c. II is due to micturition
d. II explains the pressure-volume graph when micturition fails to happen

Ans. b. Ib is due to Laplace law

13. The following image shows which of the following types of signaling?

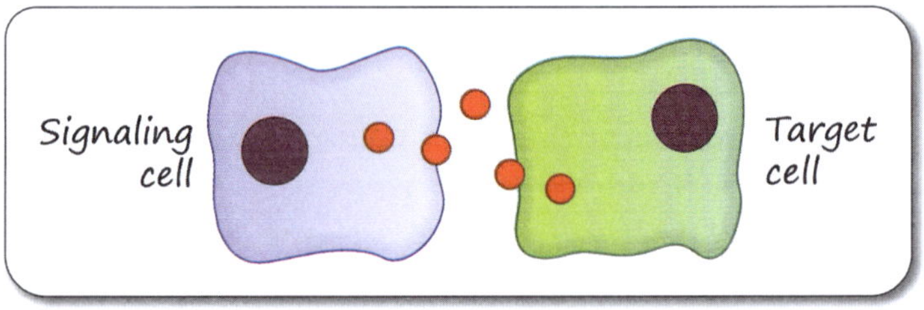

a. Paracrine
b. Autocrine
c. Endocrine
d. Merocrine

Ans. a. Paracrine

14. A person sleeps on one arm and experiences paresis in the morning but no numbness. Which of the following is the best explanation for it?

a. C fibers are more sensitive to pressure than A fibers
b. A fibers are more sensitive to hypoxia than B fibers
c. A fibers are more susceptible to pressure changes than C fibers
d. A fibers are more susceptible to hypoxia than C fibers

Ans. c. A fibers are more susceptible to pressure changes than C fibers

NEET PG 2021

15. A body fluid sample is being studied and has Na 10 mEq/L, K 140 mEq/L, Cl 4 mEq/L. Identify the fluid compartment.
   a. Interstitial
   b. ICF
   c. ECF
   d. Plasma

Ans. b. ICF

16. Beta 2 receptor action leading to hyperglycemia/hypoglycemia is mediated by which of the following enzymes?
   a. Adenylyl cyclase
   b. Guanylyl cyclase
   c. Phospholipase C
   d. Phospholipase A2

Ans. a. Adenylyl cyclase

17. A 30-year-old man weighing 70 kg had a sodium level of 120 mEq/L. Calculate the sodium deficit.
   a. 280
   b. 480
   c. 840
   d. 1400

Ans. c. 840

18. A child with loose stools for 1 day presented to your OPD. On examination, the signs of dehydration were present and the child was given ORS. It facilitates glucose absorption through which of the following receptors?
   a. SGLT1
   b. SGLT2
   c. GLUT4
   d. Na-Ca transporter

Ans. a. SGLT1

19. A chronic alcoholic patient presented with increasing abdominal girth. On examination, shifting dullness was present and the liver span was less than 7 cm. Histopathological examination revealed the presence of intracytoplasmic eosinophilic inclusions in hepatocytes. What is the content of these inclusions?
   a. Intermediate filaments
   b. Actin
   c. Microtubules
   d. Fibronectin

Ans. a. Intermediate filaments

INI-CET NOVEMBER 2023

20. What is the mechanism by which the calcium levels are increased by Parathormone (PTH)?
   a. Increase osteoclast activity
   b. Increase osteoclast activity and reduced excretion from kidney
   c. Rapid release of Ca from the osteoblast
   d. Increase osteoblast activity

Ans. b. Increase osteoclast activity and reduced excretion from kidney

21. Which of the following is responsible for the upstroke of sinoatrial nodal potential?
   a. Sodium influx via voltage gated sodium channels
   b. Sodium influx by HCN channels
   c. Potassium efflux
   d. Calcium currents only

Ans. d. Calcium currents only

22. Intrafusal muscle spindle fibers are innervated by which nerve fibers?
   a. Gamma
   b. Delta
   c. Alpha
   d. Beta

Ans. a. Gamma

23. Which of the following is incorrect regarding the baroreceptors in the carotid sinus?
   a. Baroreceptors need the support of separate electromechanical transducers
   b. Baroreceptors express several non-selective cation channels
   c. Baroreceptors are unbranched myelinated fibers of nerve IX
   d. Pressure sensors are deep in the smooth muscle layer

Ans. d. Pressure sensors are deep in the smooth muscle layer

24. Repolarization in nerve action potential is due to?
   a. Sodium influx
   b. Potassium influx
   c. Calcium influx
   d. Potassium efflux

Ans. d. Potassium efflux

25. Which sodium transporters are present maximally in the early part of the PCT?
   i. Na-K-ATPase
   ii. Na-glucose cotransporter
   iii. Na-H antiporter
   iv. Na-HCO_3 symporter
   a. ii, iii
   b. i, ii, iii
   c. i, iv
   d. iii, iv

Ans. b. i, ii, iii

26. Which of the following is responsible for bradycardia following CO_2 insufflation during laparoscopic surgery?
   a. Vascular injury
   b. Air embolism
   c. Peritoneal stretch
   d. Decreased afterload

Ans. c. Peritoneal stretch

27. Insulin independent glucose transporter is present in all of the following; except:
   a. Brain b. RBC
   c. Pancreas d. Adipose tissue

Ans. d. Adipose tissue

INI-CET MAY 2023

28. Hypoxia due to reduced oxygen content is seen in?
   a. Hypoxic hypoxia b. Anemic hypoxia
   c. Histotoxic hypoxia d. Stagnant hypoxia

Ans. b. Anemic hypoxia

29. Assertion: RMP depends on proteins and phosphate ions.
   Reason: Diffusion potential can be calculated using Nernst Equation.
   a. Both true, reason is explanation
   b. Both true, reason is not the explanation
   c. Assertion true
   d. Reason true

Ans. b. Both true, reason is not the explanation

30. Increase in BP at the beginning of Valsalva is due to?
   a. Increase in intrathoracic pressure adds to left ventricular pressure
   b. Increase in intrathoracic pressure adds to aortic pressure
   c. Increase in left atrial pressure
   d. Increase in left ventricular volume

Ans. b. Increase in intrathoracic pressure adds to aortic pressure

31. Pressure measured at upper airway becomes zero when measured at which volume/capacity?
   a. Inspiratory capacity
   b. Functional residual capacity
   c. Residual volume
   d. Total lung capacity

Ans. b. Functional residual capacity

32. Which of the following hormone acts via JAK-STAT pathway?
   a. Calcitonin b. Vasopressin
   c. Aldosterone d. Leptin

Ans. d. Leptin

33. Cells prolific in smooth endoplasmic reticulum secrete:
   a. Eicosanoid hormones b. Steroid hormones
   c. Amine hormones d. Peptide hormones

Ans. b. Steroid hormones

34. Arrange the following bands in sarcomere in sequence from periphery to center:
   a. Z line b. M line
   c. A band d. H zone

Ans. a, c, d, b

35. Which of the following is true about skeletal muscle?
   a. Extracellular Ca is not important for contraction
   b. Ca is mainly released from mitochondria
   c. Ca is released from sarcoplasmic reticulum
   d. Voltage gated Ca channel on sarcolemma has no role in EC coupling

Ans. c. Ca is released from sarcoplasmic reticulum

36. Our body can identify toxic substances by the recognition of bitter taste. This bitter taste is due to which component?
   a. Alkaloids
   b. Amino acids
   c. Hydrogen ions
   d. Aldehyde

Ans. a. Alkaloids

37. Which of the following is responsible for fetal heart acceleration?
   a. Atrial natriuretic peptide
   b. Carotid body chemoreceptors
   c. Autonomic brain stem regulation
   d. Aortic baroreceptors

Ans. b. Carotid body chemoreceptors

38. Which of the following statement is false about male sexual development?
   a. Dihydrotestosterone leads to the development of secondary sexual characters and external genitalia
   b. Wolffian duct develops into Epididymis and vas deferens on either side of the body
   c. Mullerian inhibiting substance inhibits Mullerian duct
   d. At 8th week, fetus is bipotential

Ans. d. At 8th week, fetus is bipotential

39. Which of the following are incorrectly paired?
   a. Gastrin - G cells, Antrum
   b. Secretin - S cells, Duodenum
   c. CCK - I cells, Duodenum and jejunum
   d. Motilin- M cells, Duodenum and Jejunum

Ans. d. Motilin- M cells, Duodenum and Jejunum

40. Windkessel effect is shown by all of the following; except:
   a. Renal artery
   b. Aorta
   c. Carotid artery
   d. Radial artery

Ans. d. Radial artery

41. Arrange the following neuroanatomical structures from receptor to cerebral cortex:
   a. Spiral ganglion
   b. Cochlear nucleus
   c. Inferior Colliculus
   d. Olivary Nucleus
   e. Medial geniculate body

Ans. a, b, d, c, e

INI-CET NOVEMBER 2022

42. Ventricular action potential sequence order?
   a. Opening of voltage-gated sodium channels
   b. Transient outward flow of potassium
   c. Opening of voltage-gated calcium channels
   d. Repolarizing K^+ currents

Ans. a, b, c, d

43. Oxygen dissociation curve of rectangular hyperbola is for:
   a. Methemoglobin
   b. Carboxyhemoglobin
   c. Fetal hemoglobin
   d. Myoglobin

Ans. d. Myoglobin

44. How do you calculate cerebral perfusion pressure?
   a. MAP-ICP
   b. SBP - ICP
   c. MAP/ICP
   d. SBP + ICP

Ans. a. MAP-ICP

45. Fluid leaving the PCT in the absence of ADH is:
   a. Isotonic
   b. Hypotonic
   c. Hypertonic
   d. Depends on fluid intake

Ans. a. Isotonic

46. Match the following molecules with their carriers in plasma:

Transporter-	Organic substance-
1. Prealbumin	a. Thyroxine
2. Albumin	b. Fatty acid
3. Haptoglobin	c. Hemoglobin
4. Hemopexin	d. Heme

Ans. 1-a, 2-b, 3-c, 4-d

47. **Which among the following organs have least arteriovenous pressure difference?**
   a. Brain
   b. Skin
   c. Liver
   d. Kidney

Ans. d. Kidney

48. **How does 2, 3 BPG decrease the affinity of hemoglobin to oxygen?**
   a. Binds to alpha chain
   b. Binds to beta chain
   c. Binds to gamma chain
   d. Binds to both alpha and beta chains

Ans. b. Binds to beta chain

49. **Cardiac output can be calculated from:**
   a. ECHO
   b. Ventilation-perfusion scan
   c. Thermodilution
   d. Fick's principle

Ans. a, c, d

50. **Match the following structures with their markers:**

a. Mitochondria (inner membrane)	1. Catalase
b. Endoplasmic Reticulum	2. Galactosyl transferase
c. Golgi body	3. Glucose 6 Phosphatase
d. Peroxisomes	4. ATP synthase

Ans. a-4, b-3, c-2, d-1

51. **The primary second messenger involved in the contraction of ciliary muscle during focusing on near object is:**
   a. cAMP
   b. cGMP
   c. IP3
   d. Na inflow through a channel

Ans. c. IP3

52. **Macula densa is made of specialized cells located at:**
   a. Junction of thick descending limb and DCT
   b. Junction of thick descending limb and PCT
   c. Junction of thick ascending limb and DCT
   d. Junction of DCT and collecting duct

Ans. c. Junction of thick ascending limb and DCT

53. **A woman has vomiting whenever she eats spicy food. Arrange the sequence of events during vomiting.**
   a. Contraction of diaphragm and abdominal muscles
   b. Inspiration against closed glottis
   c. LES opens and UES opens
   d. Reverse peristalsis in small intestine

Ans. b, d, a, c

54. **Value of oncotic pressure of tissue is:**
   a. 12 mm Hg b. 15 mm Hg
   c. 25 mm Hg d. 5 mm Hg

Ans. d. 5 mm Hg

INI-CET MAY 2022

55. **Which of the following leads to detachment of myosin head from the actin?**
   a. Release of ADP and Pi
   b. Attachment of ATP on myosin head
   c. Attachment of ATP on actin
   d. Release of ADP from actin

Ans. b. Attachment of ATP on myosin head

56. **Countercurrent mechanism seen in**
   1. Kidney 2. Skin
   3. Intestine 4. Testes
   a. 1, 2, 3, 4 b. 1, 2
   c. 1, 2, 3 d. 2, 3

Ans. a. 1, 2, 3, 4

57. Identify the correctly matched pair:
1. Simple diffusion – oxygen
2. Facilitated diffusion – calcium ATPase
3. Sodium potassium ATPase- secondary active transport
4. SGLT- primary active transport

a. 1 b. 2
c. 3 d. 4

Ans. a. 1

58. Which of the following acts by increasing phospholipase C?
a. Gs b. Gi
c. Gt d. Gq

Ans. d. Gq

59. All of the following are seen as a part of acclimatization to high altitude; except:
a. Hyperventilation
b. Metabolic acidosis
c. Pulmonary vasoconstriction
d. Respiratory alkalosis

Ans. b. Metabolic acidosis

INI-CET NOVEMBER 2021

60. Sodium iodide symporter is present in all of the following; except:
a. Thyroid gland b. Pituitary gland
c. Placenta d. Salivary gland

Ans. b. Pituitary gland

61. A skeletal muscle has latent period, contraction period and relaxation period of 10s, 40s and 50s respectively. Calculate the tetanizing frequency.
a. 100 b. 25
c. 50 d. 0

Ans. b. 25

62. Which of the following waves corresponds to an isovolumetric contraction in JVP?
a. a b. c
c. v d. x

Ans. b. c

63. Lesion in which lobe will lead to impairment of hand-eye coordination?
a. Temporal lobe b. Parietal lobe
c. Occipital lobe d. Frontal lobe

Ans. b. Parietal lobe

64. Right shift of oxygen dissociation curve is seen in all of the following; except:
a. Acidosis
b. Increased 2, 3 DPG levels
c. Increased HbF levels
d. Increased CO_2 concentration

Ans. c. Increased HbF levels

65. All of the following increases gastric acid secretion; except:
a. Serotonin
b. Acetylcholine
c. Histamine
d. Gastrin

Ans. a. Serotonin

66. Pacinian corpuscle is stimulated by which of the following?
a. Pressure
b. Touch
c. Cold temperature
d. Hot temperature

Ans. a. Pressure

67. A patient came with hypoxemia and a normal arterial alveolar oxygen gradient. What can be the cause?
a. Hypoventilation
b. Right to left shunt
c. Thickened basement membrane
d. Alveolar membrane damage

Ans. a. Hypoventilation

68. Which among the following has the highest airway resistance?
a. Small-sized bronchioles
b. Respiratory bronchioles
c. Alveolar duct
d. Bronchus

Ans. d. Bronchus

69. All of the following ions have decreased concentration on the luminal side of PCT; except:
 a. Bicarbonate
 b. Chloride
 c. Glucose
 d. Amino acids

Ans. b. Chloride

70. What will happen to the pressure-volume curve when the contractility of the heart changes?
 a. End diastolic volume and pressure curve shift to left without change in slope
 b. End systolic volume and pressure curve shift to right without change in slope.
 c. Slope changes in EDV and pressure curve
 d. Slope changes in ESV and pressure curve

Ans. d. Slope changes in ESV and pressure curve

INI-CET JULY 2021

71. Which of the following is not involved in renal autoregulation?
 a. Tubuloglomerular feedback
 b. Myogenic reflex
 c. Renin-angiotensin system
 d. Renal sympathetic system fibers

Ans. d. Renal sympathetic system fibers

72. The formula for urea clearance is UxV/P, where U is:
 a. Urine volume
 b. Serum urea in mg /100 mL
 c. Urine urea in g/24h
 d. Urine urea in mg/mL

Ans. d. Urine urea in mg/mL

73. The relaxation of the intestinal segment distal to the segment with the bolus of food during peristalsis is because of?
 a. VIP
 b. Substance P
 c. Dopamine from adrenergic fibers
 d. Acetylcholine from myenteric fibers

Ans. a. VIP

74. A patient presented with severe watery diarrhea resembling that of rice gruel stool. Damage of which structure is likely to have resulted in this diarrhea?
 a. Zona occludens
 b. Gap junction
 c. Adherent junction
 d. Hemidesmosomes

Ans. a. Zona occludens

75. Beta hCG is structurally similar to which biochemical moiety?
 a. LH
 b. FSH
 c. ACTH
 d. Oxytocin

Ans. a. LH

76. What is the duration of short-term memory?
 a. 3-6 hours
 b. 12-18 hours
 c. 30-300 seconds
 d. 3-4 seconds

Ans. c. 30-300 seconds

77. The stroke volume depends on end-diastolic volume. This is best represented as:
 a. Length-force relationship
 b. Length-velocity relationship
 c. Length-tension relationship
 d. Length-viscosity relationship

Ans. c. Length-tension relationship

78. Which of the following ions in the thick ascending limb of the loop of Henle is responsible for the resorption of divalent ions?
 a. H^+
 b. HCO_3^-
 c. K^+
 d. Na^+

Ans. c. K^+

79. Which of the following sensory receptors are responsible for tactile discrimination?
 a. Merkel disc
 b. Ruffini end organ
 c. Pacinian corpuscle
 d. Meissner's corpuscle

Ans. d. Meissner's corpuscle

FMGE JANUARY 2024

80. Which of the following interferes with iron absorption?
   a. Amla juice b. Lemon juice
   c. Tea d. Sprouts

Ans. c. Tea

81. Which of the following is associated with cardiac tamponade?
   a. Absent Y descent b. Absent X descent
   c. Cannon a wave d. Absent a wave

Ans. a. Absent Y descent

82. Temperature regulating center is located in:
   a. Amygdala b. Hippocampus
   c. Hypothalamus d. Prefrontal cortex

Ans. c. Hypothalamus

83. Dynein is a/an:
   a. Transport protein
   b. Cell membrane protein
   c. Adherent protein
   d. Molecular motor

Ans. d. Molecular motor

84. Patient can speak fluently but lacks meaning and understanding. This type of aphasia is:
   a. Broca's aphasia
   b. Wernicke's aphasia
   c. Conduction aphasia
   d. Anomic aphasia

Ans. b. Wernicke's aphasia

85. Skeletal muscle, heart, adipose tissue have which type of GLUT?
   a. GLUT 1 b. GLUT 2
   c. GLUT 3 d. GLUT 4

Ans. d. GLUT 4

86. Central veins have which type of cells in the center?
   a. Lymphocytes b. Neutrophils
   c. Macrophages d. RBCs

Ans. d. RBCs

87. Identify the marked volume/capacity.

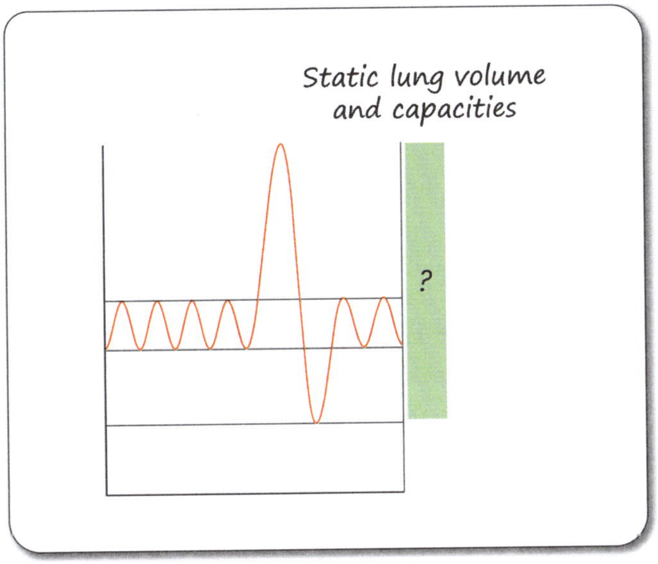

   a. Functional residual capacity
   b. Tidal volume
   c. Vital capacity
   d. Total lung capacity

Ans. c. Vital capacity

FMGE JANUARY 2023

88. Clotting factor of extrinsic pathway is:
   a. Factor IX
   b. Factor VIII
   c. Factor XII
   d. Factor VII

Ans. d. Factor VII

89. Hemoglobin with iron in ferric form is called:
   a. Fetal hemoglobin
   b. Methemoglobin
   c. HbS
   d. Adult hemoglobin

Ans. b. Methemoglobin

90. Serum osmolarity is determined primarily by:
   a. Bicarbonate
   b. Potassium
   c. Hydrogen ions
   d. Sodium

Ans. d. Sodium

91. **Large V wave in JVP is seen in:**
   a. Tricuspid regurgitation
   b. Atrial fibrillation
   c. Aortic regurgitation
   d. Tricuspid stenosis

Ans. a. Tricuspid regurgitation

92. **Which of the following is true regarding creatinine clearance?**
   a. Equal to renal plasma flow
   b. Less than inulin clearance
   c. Equal to inulin clearance
   d. More than inulin clearance

Ans. d. More than inulin clearance

93. **The first heart sound coincides with:**
   a. Aortic ejection
   b. Isovolumic relaxation
   c. Isovolumic contraction
   d. Rapid filling

Ans. c. Isovolumic contraction

94. **Hypoxia in high altitude is due to:**
   a. High partial pressure of CO_2
   b. Low partial pressure of CO_2
   c. High partial pressure of O_2
   d. Low partial pressure of O_2

Ans. d. Low partial pressure of O_2

95. **Orexigenic hormone is:**
   a. Cholecystokinin
   b. Leptin
   c. Ghrelin
   d. Melanocyte stimulating hormone

Ans. c. Ghrelin

96. **Which of the following is true about glomerular filtration rate (GFR)?**
   a. Sympathetic stimulation increases GFR
   b. Afferent arteriole constriction increases GFR
   c. Increase in renal plasma flow increases GFR
   d. Decrease in renal plasma flow increases GFR

Ans. c. Increase in renal plasma flow increases GFR

FMGE JULY 2023

97. **Where is the location of thyroid hormone receptor?**
   a. Transmembrane receptor
   b. Nuclear receptor
   c. Cytoplasmic receptor
   d. G protein coupled receptor

Ans. b. Nuclear receptor

98. **Which of the following statement is correct regarding phase Ib of cystometrogram?**

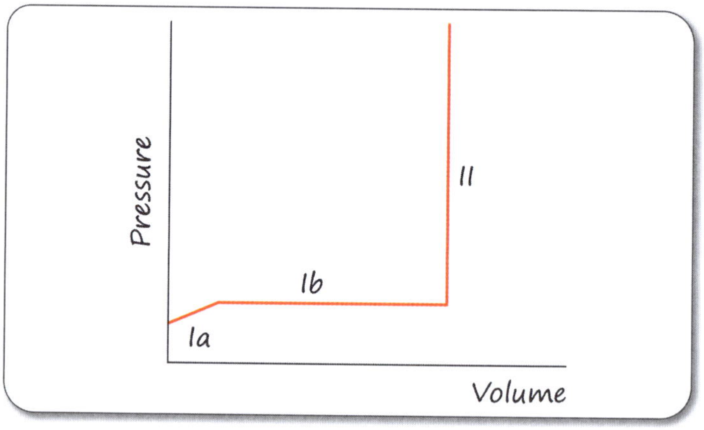

   a. Due to elasticity of bladder
   b. Due to plasticity of bladder
   c. Contractility of bladder
   d. Micturition starts at phase Ib

Ans. b. Due to plasticity of bladder

99. **Negative feedback regulation for follicle stimulating hormone and luteinizing hormone are?**
   a. Testosterone and inhibin
   b. Testosterone and DHEA
   c. Testosterone and estrogen
   d. Inhibin and testosterone

Ans. d. Inhibin and testosterone

100. **Hypotension, bradycardia and apnea after injection of irritant substance is:**
   a. Cushing reflex
   b. Bainbridge reflex
   c. Bezold-Jarisch reflex
   d. Marey's law

Ans. c. Bezold-Jarisch reflex

101. In a patient with hypotension, neck vein distension and muffled heart sounds, which of the following is expected?
   a. Absent Y descent
   b. Absent X descent
   c. Cannon a wave
   d. Absent a wave

Ans. a. Absent Y descent

102. ECG finding in Wolff-Parkinson-White syndrome is:
   a. Wide QRS
   b. Diminished AV delay
   c. Prolong PR interval
   d. Short QRS

Ans. a. Wide QRS

103. GLUT-2 is present in:
   a. Kidney
   b. Brain
   c. Liver
   d. Intestine

Ans. c. Liver

104. All of the following are seen during acclimatization in high altitude; except:
   a. Hypoventilation
   b. Increase in myoglobin
   c. Increase in hemoglobin
   d. Polycythemia

Ans. a. Hypoventilation

105. Hormone responsible for galactokinesis is:
   a. Vasopressin
   b. Insulin
   c. Aldosterone
   d. Oxytocin

Ans. d. Oxytocin

106. Which of the following inhibits insulin secretion?
   a. Gastric inhibitory peptide
   b. Acetylcholine
   c. Epinephrine
   d. Glucagon

Ans. c. Epinephrine

107. Which of the following is not a function of intestinal epithelium?
   a. Absorption of ions
   b. Bile salt secretion
   c. Formation of digestive enzymes
   d. Mucus secretion

Ans. b. Bile salt secretion

108. Nerve fiber responsible for intense superficial pain is:
   a. A alpha
   b. C
   c. A delta
   d. A beta

Ans. c. A delta

FMGE JUNE 2022

109. Delivery on uterine contraction is similar to:
   a. Water retention by ADH
   b. Milk ejection by oxytocin
   c. Vasoconstriction by norepinephrine
   d. Increase in food intake by ghrelin

Ans. b. Milk ejection by oxytocin

110. Which of the following is not done by estrogen?
   a. Cervical mucus secretion
   b. Menstruation
   c. Vaginal cornification
   d. Pubic and axillary hair growth

Ans. d. Pubic and axillary hair growth

111. Mechanism of action of atrial natriuretic peptide is through:
   a. cAMP
   b. cGMP
   c. IP3-DAG
   d. JAK STAT

Ans. b. cGMP

112. Affinity of carbon monoxide to hemoglobin in comparison to oxygen is:
   a. 150
   b. 175
   c. 250
   d. 4

Ans. c. 250

113. Second messenger involved in gastric secretion is:
   a. cAMP
   b. cGMP
   c. Janus Kinase
   d. Tyrosine kinase

Ans. a. cAMP

114. Cramps in breast in breastfeeding are due to:
   a. Estrogen
   b. Prolactin
   c. Progesterone
   d. Oxytocin

Ans. d. Oxytocin

115. Insulin acts on glucose metabolism by?
a. Increase glucose absorption from intestine
b. Increase glucose reabsorption from renal tubules
c. Increase facilitated diffusion of glucose
d. Decrease permeability of glucose across cell membrane

Ans. c. Increase facilitated diffusion of glucose

116. If the diameter of a vessel is reduced by 1/3rd, then how much resistance will increase?
a. 9 times
b. 18 times
c. 81 times
d. 27 times

Ans. c. 81 times

117. Secretory diarrhea is seen in:
a. Insulinoma
b. Glucagonoma
c. VIPoma
d. Zollinger-Ellison syndrome

Ans. c. VIPoma

118. Conversion of T_4 to T_3 in periphery is done by:
a. Deiodinase I
b. Deiodinase II
c. Deiodinase III
d. Deiodinase IV

Ans. a. Deiodinase I

FMGE DECEMBER 2021

119. Oxygen dissociation is shifted to left in:
a. Hypoxia
b. Hypercarbia
c. Alkalosis
d. Increase in 2, 3 DPG

Ans. c. Alkalosis

120. Cell organelle involved in killing bacteria and virus is:
a. Peroxisomes
b. Golgi apparatus
c. Nucleus
d. Lysosomes

Ans. d. Lysosomes

121. After ileal and partial jejunal resection, the patient will have:
a. Gastric ulcer
b. Constipation
c. Vitamin B_{12} deficiency
d. Folate deficiency

Ans. c. Vitamin B_{12} deficiency

122. Contralateral loss of pain and temperature sensation is seen in:
a. Wallenberg syndrome
b. Werner syndrome
c. Pearson syndrome
d. Brown-Sequard Syndrome

Ans. d. Brown-Sequard syndrome

FMGE JUNE 2021

123. Reflex responsible for tachycardia during right atrial distension is:
a. Cushing reflex
b. Bainbridge reflex
c. Bezold-Jarisch reflex
d. Marey's law

Ans. b. Bainbridge reflex

124. As filtrate passes through proximal convoluted tubule, the concentration of all of the following decreases; except:
a. Bicarbonate
b. Glucose
c. Chloride
d. Amino acids

Ans. c. Chloride

125. Why hemoglobin cannot pass through glomerulus?

a. Gets attracted to positive charge on basement membrane
b. Large protein bounded to another protein
c. Both a and b
d. Small protein

Ans. b. Large protein bounded to another protein

126. Following injury, a patient is extremely curious and tries touching everything. He even tried to eat the plates. Where is the lesion?

a. Cingulate gyrus
b. Occipital lobe
c. Hypothalamus
d. Amygdala

Ans. d. Amygdala

127. Surfactant is secreted by:

a. Alveolar macrophages
b. Clara cells
c. Type I pneumocytes
d. Type II pneumocytes

Ans. d. Type II pneumocytes

128. Which hormone regulates serum calcium levels?

a. Calcitonin
b. Vitamin D
c. Parathormone
d. All of the above

Ans. d. All of the above

129. Corticospinal tract crosses at:

a. Upper medulla
b. Lower medulla
c. Pons
d. Midbrain

Ans. b. Lower medulla

Notes